W9-CEH-689

Getting that Medical Job

Secrets for Success

Getting that Medical Job

Secrets for Success

Colin J. Mumford

BMedSci, BM, BS, DM, FRCP, FRCPEdin, Dip IMC RCSEd
Consultant Neurologist
Department of Clinical Neurosciences
Western General Hospital
Edinburgh

Suvankar Pal

BSc MB BS MRCP(UK) MD(Res)
Registrar in Neurology
Department of Clinical Neurosciences
Western General Hospital
Edinburgh

THIRD EDITION

⊛ WILEY-BLACKWELL

A John Wiley & Sons, Ltd., Publication

This edition first published 2011 © 2011 by Colin J. Mumford and Suvankar Pal

Blackwell Publishing was acquired by John Wiley & Sons in February 2007. Blackwell's publishing program has been merged with Wiley's global Scientific, Technical and Medical business to form Wiley-Blackwell.

Registered office: John Wiley & Sons, Ltd, The Atrium, Southern Gate, Chichester, West Sussex, PO19 8SQ, UK

Editorial offices: 9600 Garsington Road, Oxford, OX4 2DQ, UK
              The Atrium, Southern Gate, Chichester, West Sussex, PO19 8SQ, UK
              111 River Street, Hoboken, NJ 07030-5774, USA

For details of our global editorial offices, for customer services and for information about how to apply for permission to reuse the copyright material in this book please see our website at www.wiley.com/wiley-blackwell

Library of Congress Cataloging-in-Publication Data

Mumford, Colin John.
  Getting that medical job : secrets for success/Colin J. Mumford, Suvankar Pal. – 3rd ed.
    p. ; cm.
  Rev. ed. of: The medical job interview/Colin J. Mumford. 2nd ed. 2005.
  Includes bibliographical references and index.
  ISBN 978-1-4443-3488-3 (pbk. : alk. paper)   1. Medicine–Vocational guidance–Great Britain.   2. Employment interviewing–Great Britain.   3. Physicians–Employment–Great Britain. I. Pal, Suvankar. II. Mumford, Colin John. Medical job interview.
III. Title.
  [DNLM: 1. Interviews as Topic–Great Britain.   2. Job Application–Great Britain.
3. Physicians–Great Britain. W 21]
  R690.M785 2011
  610.690941–dc22

                                                2010047395

A catalogue record for this book is available from the British Library.

Set in 9/12 pt Palatino by Aptara® Inc., New Delhi, India
Printed and bound in Malaysia by Vivar Printing Sdn Bhd

1 2011

CONTENTS

Contents

PREFACE

I wrote the first edition of this book about 5 years after appointment to a consultant post in a Scottish teaching hospital. I had a fresh memory of all my interviews for the 'training grade' posts, and I was regularly invited to sit on panels for interview of both junior hospital doctors and applicants for consultant posts. At that stage it was pretty clear to me what a candidate needed to do in order to be successful – or at least have a very good chance of success – at every level.

But times change, and so do interview processes. Even when the second edition was produced in 2005, neither I nor the publishers could have foreseen the mayhem that was about to descend in the form of 'Modernising Medical Careers' – a bizarre and unreliable system of appointment imposed on the medical profession by faceless individuals in the UK Department of Health, with the acquiescence of some very senior clinicians who really ought to have known better.

Thankfully, the weight of protest that ensued made Whitehall mandarins see sense, and many of the most galling aspects of the 'MMC' process have been removed. Some though, remain, and interview candidates still have to contend with online application processes, requirements to justify an application for a given post in fewer than a couple of hundred words, national interviews held at a single centre on just 1 day in the year, and the possibility of being interviewed for a post in a given location by an individual who themselves may never have set foot in the hospital to which the candidate might be appointed.

Changes like this mean that senior doctors like me are a bit 'out of the loop' when it comes to being really savvy about what is needed to triumph in the interview process in its present form. So for the third edition of this book I had to get help. I needed to find a co-author who was fully up to speed with every aspect of the 'new look' medical interview process, and who had clearly shown himself to be a stellar performer when being interviewed. The obvious candidate was identified at the end of a busy outpatient clinic: my own registrar, Dr Suvankar Pal.

Suvankar has handled the lion's share of work needed for the preparation of this third edition. He has grilled junior trainees regarding their success or failure with online applications, he has made them transcribe memories of questions posed and their own answers proffered at national interviews, and has made them spill the beans in terms of confessing their glaring errors and blunders when they recall their own performances. This diligent fact-finding has meant that Suvankar has been able to produce a great deal of new material for this book, with many descriptions of successful and less successful answers to questions, both online and in spoken interviews. I am enormously grateful to Suvankar for all his tireless work.

As well as the arrival of a second author, readers will also note that there are several new chapters in this third edition, including specific advice on strategies to use in specialist registrar interviews and academic interviews, many word-for-word records of good and bad answers to real questions, and more information on how to approach the first consultant-level interview.

I think the changes represent a big improvement over the first and second editions of this book. Let's see if you agree.

Colin Mumford
Edinburgh

ACKNOWLEDGEMENTS

A large number of good friends helped me in the preparation of the second edition of this book, and the same individuals were pestered to help with this third edition. Suggestions for new content, and comments on old, came from senior hospital doctors, junior doctors in training, secondary school teachers, representatives of the pharmaceutical industry and members of some of the more interesting parts of the British Civil Service. To all of these people I would like to offer enormous thanks. The team at Wiley-Blackwell had excellent ideas to improve the content for this third edition, and they have my gratitude too.

Finally a number of junior colleagues spent some time recalling their own interview experiences, both good and bad, and some have very generously allowed their actual words to be reproduced in this book. This was 'above and beyond' the call of duty.

NOTE FOR WOULD-BE MEDICAL STUDENTS

The first two editions of this book were written for final-year medical students and junior hospital doctors in training. They were never really intended to be a guide to help sixth-formers seeking a place at medical school. Nevertheless, quite a large number of copies of the first and second editions were sold to A-level candidates, and I suspect some of the suggestions that I made were applicable to the process of gaining entry into university. This still holds true for this third edition of the work. Certainly, I think many of the ideas regarding 'pre-interview groundwork' could be utilised by the enthusiastic sixth-former wanting to make sure that they receive a good offer from their first-choice medical school.

INTRODUCTION

chapter 1

The aim of this short book is simple. It is to make sure that you're successful in your next medical job interview. It is quite possible to be a wonderful medical student or doctor with encyclopaedic knowledge of medical conditions, first-class clinical skills and a terrific rapport with all your patients, but if you can't perform well in the job interviews then you will get nowhere. This book sets out to give you tips that will be equally relevant, whether you are a final-year medical student applying for your first house job, i.e to become an 'FY1', an 'FY2' (the new name for a senior house officer) trying to break through onto the specialist registrar career ladder, or if you are reaching the end of your specialist registrar training and are seeking appointment to your first consultant post.

Note that virtually all that is contained in this book is relevant to the UK system of medical training. Graduates in Ireland

Getting that Medical Job: Secrets for Success, 3rd edition. © Colin J. Mumford and Suvankar Pal. Published 2011 by Blackwell Publishing Ltd.

and Western Europe may find some of the information useful. But we must leave it up to colleagues in the USA and Canada to decide whether they feel that this 'very British approach' is of any benefit in winning over interview panels in North America! Readers outside the United Kingdom may be surprised to learn that face-to-face interviews for the very junior hospital posts in Britain no longer occur. Instead, much is done via an online process, so the chance for candidates to excel in their oral interview performance has been lost. However, in some countries where this book is used, these lower level interviews still take place, and we have recognised that fact in many of the following chapters, retaining comments on optimal strategies for junior-level interviews where relevant.

Even British graduates need to appreciate that we are giving advice from the point of view of hospital doctors. I am a hospital consultant who has worked his way up through the British *hospital* medical career ladder. My new co-author is also progressing up the specialty training route. A rather different emphasis and series of tricks are needed in breaking into the world of general practice. All the same, some of the tips that we give here may at least be starters for someone approaching an interview to be a registrar in general practice, or even seeking appointment to their first post as principal in GP-land.

The astonishing thing about most British medical graduates is that although they prepare in enormous detail for clinical medical school exams and for postgraduate diplomas, such as the MRCP(UK), MRCOG, FRCS and so on, most of them put relatively little thought into planning their strategy for handling a medical job interview. This is a grave error since there is no doubt that good interview technique can be learned. Some people begin their careers already good at it, but others are so bad that they could only be described as appalling in an interview, and it is this latter group who most need to do their homework prior to facing an interview panel!

Throughout this book we've tended to use the word 'he' when, of course, we mean 'he or she'. Writing 'he or she' every time becomes clumsy.

If you have suggestions for future editions of this book, please email **medicalstudent@wiley.co.uk.**

CHOOSING THE SPECIALTY THAT'S RIGHT FOR YOU

chapter 2

Although this book is primarily aimed at ensuring your success in the interview process, if you are a final year student or junior doctor at the start of your postgraduate training, then it is worth pausing to think about which subject you're going to choose to become your life-long work. Deciding which specialty to apply for can seem overwhelming. With the advent of 'run-through' training, applications made less than 2 years after graduating from medical school may potentially define the next 4 decades of a medical career! Whilst narrowing down the choices can be daunting, time spent reflecting on your own attributes, career ambitions and researching what the different specialties have to offer is a must and can be surprisingly rewarding. Forming clear ideas in your own mind about why you are choosing a particular specialty will stand you in good stead for completing application form answers and shining at the interview. Initial interest and experience in a particular specialty may stem from medical school. If you're lucky, you may have gained further experience during an overseas elective, special study modules and

Getting that Medical Job: Secrets for Success, 3rd edition. © Colin J. Mumford and Suvankar Pal. Published 2011 by Blackwell Publishing Ltd.

placements, as a foundation year or junior specialty doctor. This may not always be possible though, and there are many specialties such as medical microbiology, chemical pathology and public health where exposure at junior level is limited and other specialties such as tropical medicine, allergy and audiological medicine which you may not even have realised existed!

So whom to ask and where to look? The first thing to be aware of is the very large number of specialties available which are broadly divided into: (1) Themed core specialties (including emergency medicine and anaesthesia), (2) Medical specialties, (3) Surgical specialties, (4) Psychiatry and (5) Run-through specialties. The latter are specialties to which commitment must be made at a very early stage, since a 'one track' training programme exists with very little scope to change to a different specialty along the course. This route currently includes both general practice and paediatrics.

THEMED CORE SPECIALTIES

- Acute care common stem (ACCS)
- Acute medicine
- Anaesthesia
- Emergency medicine

MEDICAL SPECIALTIES

- Core medical training
- Acute medicine
- Allergy
- Audiological medicine
- Cardiology
- Clinical genetics
- Clinical neurophysiology
- Clinical oncology
- Clinical pharmacology and therapeutics

- Dermatology
- Endocrinology and diabetes
- Gastroenterology
- Genito-urinary medicine
- Geriatric medicine
- Haematology
- Immunology
- Infectious diseases
- Infectious diseases and medical microbiology
- Infectious diseases and virology
- Medical oncology
- Medical ophthalmology
- Neurology
- Nuclear medicine
- Occupational medicine
- Palliative medicine
- Paediatric cardiology
- Rehabilitation medicine
- Renal medicine
- Respiratory medicine
- Rheumatology
- Sports and exercise medicine
- Tropical medicine

SURGICAL SPECIALTIES

- Surgery in general (generic)
- Cardiothoracic surgery
- General surgery
- Oral and maxillofacial surgery
- Otolaryngology (ENT)
- Paediatric surgery
- Plastic surgery
- Trauma and orthopaedic surgery
- Urology

PSYCHIATRY

- Child and adolescent psychiatry
- General adult psychiatry
- Psychiatry of learning disability
- Old age psychiatry
- Forensic psychiatry
- Psychotherapy

RUN-THROUGH SPECIALTIES

- Chemical pathology
- Chemical pathology – metabolic medicine
- Clinical radiology
- General practice
- Histopathology
- Medical microbiology/virology – microbiology
- Medical microbiology/virology – virology
- Neurosurgery
- Obstetrics and gynaecology
- Ophthalmology
- Paediatrics
- Public health
- Trauma and orthopaedic surgery

Speaking to local trainees and consultants in different specialties is a good starting point. They may be able to help by arranging taster sessions and invaluable clinical shadowing experience. There is a wealth of information available on the modernising medical careers, NHS medical careers and foundation programme websites:

http://www. mmc.nhs.uk/
http://www.medicalcareers.nhs.uk/
http://www.nhscareers.nhs.uk/specialtytraining
http://www.foundationprogramme.nhs.uk/

Further information can be gained by browsing individual Royal College websites. Many of the Royal Colleges have dedicated specialty careers information days and career liaison officers:

Medicine	*http://www.rcplondon.ac.uk*
	http://www.rcpe.ac.uk/
Surgery	*http://www.rcseng.ac.uk*
	http://www.rcsed.ac.uk/
	http://www.rcpsg.ac.uk/
General practice	*http://www.rcgp.org.uk/ gp_training.aspx*
Psychiatry	*http://www.rcgp.org.uk/ www.rcpsych.ac.uk*
Obstetrics and gynaecology	*http://www.rcog.org.uk*
Emergency medicine	*http://www.collemergencymed. ac.uk/cem/*
Radiology	*http://www.rcr.ac.uk/*
Paediatrics and child health	*http://www.rcpch.ac.uk/*
Pathology	*http://www.rcpath.org/*
Anaesthetics	*http://www.rcoa.ac.uk/*
Ophthalmology	*http://www.rcophth.ac.uk/*

Many specialty-specific journals contain up-to-date information about clinical, research and service provision developments which may provide additional insight into what a career in an individual specialty may involve. Don't forget also to look at the careers section of the *British Medical Journal* which frequently contains many useful articles (*http://careers.bmj. com/*).

POINTS FOR REFLECTION

- Which specialties are you drawn to applying for and why?
- How can you gain more experience and understanding of your chosen specialty?
- Where you would ideally like to work and why?

BEFORE THE INTERVIEW

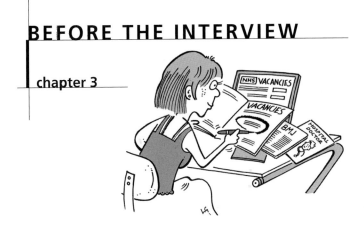

SPOTTING THE ADVERT

It sounds ridiculous, but some individuals fail at the very first hurdle in their efforts to climb the medical career ladder, and that is because they fail to spot the advert for the job which they want. This is a catastrophic mistake since the one way to guarantee not being shortlisted is failing to apply for the job in the first place. Therefore, as soon as you are even contemplating applying for your next move up the medical ladder you should be scrutinising the relevant medical press to see which adverts are appearing, scouring all the correct websites, and noting what sort of jobs are available and starting to focus your mind on the places where you would most like to work. This may mean trying to remain in your current geographical area, or you may have a particular desire to move to a different part of the country for your next job.

Getting that Medical Job: Secrets for Success, 3rd edition. © Colin J. Mumford and Suvankar Pal. Published 2011 by Blackwell Publishing Ltd.

In general terms, this task used to be made easy for British graduates because the classified section of the *British Medical Journal* listed all the available jobs coming up, and these were conveniently grouped under headings according to specialty. Now things have changed, and especially for posts at junior level, for example foundation programmes, it may be that the key positions will only be advertised on certain websites, perhaps in turn linked to specific deaneries or areas of the country. Even when the advert appears both online *and* in the *BMJ*, the electronic version may be the first to appear. Remember, also, that editors and typesetters of the *British Medical Journal* are human, and it is not uncommon to see an advert for a post, say in neurology, advertised in error under the section headed neurosurgery. Occasionally, hospitals perform rather underhand tricks, and—for reasons best known to themselves—may decide to place an advert in a not-very-obvious location, which may be in a national newspaper, in the back pages of a weekly free journal such as *Hospital Doctor* or in some other obscure site. Recent changes to the interview process, especially for training grade posts, may mean that a single advert appears for multiple jobs in the same specialty, with the locations of the posts scattered across a swathe of the country. And worse still, some specialties may only advertise once per year. Failure to spot that all-embracing advert would be a total disaster.

If you think that a post is about to be advertised yet are struggling to find the actual advertisement, then there is no harm in phoning the appropriate personnel or medical staffing department at the relevant hospital or regional postgraduate centre and asking when a particular post will be coming up. Expressing such enthusiasm at an early stage does no harm at all. But be sure that you call the right place: increasingly the placing of adverts and the administration of the interview process for posts in given specialties are being handled by the lead postgraduate dean's office for that subject. So make sure at an early stage that you know who is the 'lead dean' for your chosen specialty, and find out where he or she is based. A quick phone call to their PA may be enormously useful in letting you know the timescale for the appearance of adverts, and the schedule and venue for subsequent interviews.

One word of caution is required at this point, and that is this: some individuals are uncertain whether or not they should apply for a job. This is particularly true at the start of a medical career when people are not sure if they should hold out for 'the best' pre-registration FY1 job or whether they should accept something 'second-rate'. Sadly, the choice may be completely taken away from you anyway, as centres move to computer-based matching systems. Equally, this problem may be especially acute at the end of the medical training ladder when senior specialist registrars are uncertain whether a 'plum consultant post' is about to come up – and so they should wait for it – or whether they should go for a post which they might consider 'second division'. The way to decide whether to apply or not is to consider the situation that if you eventually get through to the medical interview and are offered the job, you need to ask yourself: 'Will I stand up, punch the air and shout "Yahooo!" if I am successful?' If you are uncertain as to whether you would be able to express such overt enthusiasm then probably you should not be applying for the post at all. This rule is there to be broken, however, and if you are genuinely not sure whether a job is the right one for you then there is no harm in putting in an application and at least going part-way through the selection process, provided that you withdraw *before* you find yourself sitting in the interview. You can withdraw, if necessary, on the morning of the interview itself, but it is a complete no–no to sit in an interview, be offered the job and then reject the offer afterwards. This goes down extremely badly with interview panels and will land you with an undesirable reputation. On the other hand, a cautious application and polite, tactful withdrawal prior to the interview, with careful explanation to the relevant consultants, will not usually cause too much upset.

'THE COMMANDO OPERATION' TO GET ON THE SHORTLIST

Once you have seen the correct advert, then the next steps to secure shortlisting for jobs at every level, used to be clear. You needed to submit the application, prepare your curriculum vitae (CV) and do various other bits of groundwork to make sure that your name got onto the shortlist. This rigorous approach used to be referred to as the 'commando operation'. Royal Marine commandos are enormously successful at what they do basically because they leave no margin for error. Every item of equipment is checked, rechecked and tested in enormous detail. The idea was that if you seriously wanted to be successful in the medical job interview then you needed to embark on a thorough, almost military, operation to make absolutely sure that you got the job. Unfortunately, old techniques to 'shade the odds in your favour' are less readily applicable to the online application processes that medical students and junior hospital doctors now face. Nevertheless they can still be worthwhile, and these techniques are certainly relevant for individuals making application for a consultant post. Like it or not, job interviews are competitive, and accordingly somehow you have to show the interview panel that you are better than everybody else that has made an application for the post. Since some jobs may receive in excess of 200 applicants, then if you sit back and wait to be shortlisted you can guarantee that you will simply be a 'face in the crowd' and you are very unlikely to be shortlisted unless there is something extraordinarily unusual about you, your online application, or your CV.

Depending on the type and grade of post that you are applying for, you will need to determine if you are completely 'locked into' an online application process, or whether there is scope to use some or all of the 'commando techniques'. There will certainly be an opportunity to do so when applying for a senior-level position. Therefore, if it looks as though you can take some steps to elevate your profile, then as soon as the appropriate job advert appears you need to be on the phone to get the relevant application forms and you need to start preparing your CV. The application forms, whether 'hard copy' or online, will almost certainly give you information about the hospital, including the names of relevant consultants and appropriate contact phone numbers and e-mail addresses.

Your immediate goal following receipt of the job description is to get yourself onto the shortlist. Other people can help you with this. Indeed, a well-judged phone call from one of your current consultants to his friend or golfing partner, who is a consultant in the relevant hospital, can work wonders. You may feel that this is somehow underhand in asking your consultant to make a phone call on your behalf, but, unfortunately, some of your competitors will have done this, and you need to make sure you are playing in the same ball game. Bear in mind that although a helpful phone call highlighting your name may significantly improve your chances of getting on to the shortlist, once you have made it onto that shortlist, you are then on your own and it is very unlikely that persuasive words from one of your senior colleagues will actually make a difference in the interview itself.

TO VISIT OR NOT TO VISIT?

Even for senior-level appointments, many candidates wonder if it is 'worthwhile' visiting the relevant hospital before the shortlist is announced. Anybody who does not visit the hospital is, in our view, significantly reducing their chance of getting placed on the shortlist. There is no doubt that a voluntary visit, made early, and made at your own expense in order to look around wards, departments, X-ray facilities, and so on—and ideally to meet one or two of the consultants—can be enormously rewarding. The progress of a whole career can be changed by 'bumping into' the relevant consultant or professor in the corridor outside his office. If you can achieve this then you are already one rung higher than all your competitors in the fight to get on to the shortlist. Be mindful of the fact that most senior consultants are very busy and do not take kindly to being interrupted in their office or being stopped whilst walking in the corridor on route to clinic. Therefore, you need to be sharp and to the point in introducing yourself to them and you should ask if there is a point 'later in the day' when you might be able to spend 5 minutes with them since you are 'most interested' in the forthcoming job on their unit. Most consultants will accept this sort of approach but will not wish to spend 5 or 10 minutes in the corridor discussing things when they, undoubtedly, will have more important things to do. However, a request to meet later in the day may be acceptable to them.

If, having 'bumped into' the relevant consultant, you find that he is still not willing to see you, then there is no reason at all why you should not go and see his secretary and ask if you might talk to him on another occasion, or whether there are a few moments at the end of the day when he will be less busy. If nothing else, you can attempt to endear yourself to the relevant secretary such that she may make a favourable comment later in the day when she is dealing with other aspects of the consultant's work.

This initial visit must not be confused with the visits that are frequently made following the publication of the short list. Many hospitals send a letter with their initial information pack saying something to the extent of 'shortlisted candidates will be invited to visit the hospital'. Frustratingly, this is now less common for junior-level appointments, when remote offices in distant deaneries may be arranging a sequence of interviews for junior appointments in several different units. But they continue at senior level, and these visits will generally be arranged and timetabled by the secretary of the most senior consultant involved. Afterwards, the hospital will reimburse you with the costs of your travel. Bear in mind that you will only have the chance of doing this once you are already on the shortlist, and therefore a visit prior to shortlisting is, in our opinion, essential to show enthusiasm and to start to set yourself apart from the crowd.

For senior-level appointments, the process of shortlisting will usually be done by the head of the relevant department to which you are applying and also by a number of his consultant colleagues. It is very unlikely that members of the hospital management will be involved in the shortlisting process, although occasionally representatives of the regional postgraduate dean may have some votes. Therefore, if you are going to make a visit prior to shortlisting, and we advise that you do, then you should concentrate solely on seeing the clinicians for whom you would be working. If the post which you are applying for is at foundation year 1 (FY1) or foundation year 2 (FY2) level, and you are given the opportunity to visit, then try to see some of the specialist registrars working on the unit as well, since you would be surprised how much exchange of ideas takes place at the end of a ward round when consultants have a habit of discussing with their registrars potential candidates for shortlisting.

Although the initial visit that we are advocating prior to shortlisting could be considered as being 'relatively informal', you need all the while to be aware of the fact that you have one goal only, and that is to convince the people whom you meet that you are the single best candidate for the forthcoming job. Accordingly, part of the process requires that you look smart, engage in appropriately focused conversation with the doctors you meet, and, above all, have a large number of spare copies of your CV to distribute. Most of the senior clinicians will not see your CV until very shortly before they are asked to produce a shortlist, and so, if your name is to be remembered, you must pull a CV out of your bag and leave it with the relevant consultant 'for his perusal once you have gone'.

Once you have returned to your base hospital following this pre-shortlisting visit, make sure that you discuss what went on with your current bosses since if they have not already telephoned their colleagues at the new hospital to put in a word on your behalf, this is the time at which you should ask them to do so.

WHOM TO SEE ONCE YOU ARE SHORTLISTED

Once the shortlist has been produced, and hopefully, has your name on it, then whether or not you previously visited, you are now absolutely obliged to go and visit the relevant hospital. Clearly, this is only going to be of use if you know the likely hospital of appointment. Sadly, some of the newer application processes carry no certainty regarding the location in which you will be working, assuming success in the interview. But if there is at least a 'probability' of the name and location of the new base, then you must go. You should not be out of pocket as a result, since in general your travel expenses for a visit at this stage will be refunded to you. Your priority, once again, is to meet with the consultants for whom you will be working, or, if a senior post, whom you will be working alongside, but bear in mind that during the interview itself there will almost certainly be some non-medical interviewers, for example a member of the hospital management or a representative of the Trust Board. Therefore, at least one of your visits must be to the chief executive of the hospital, or, if he is not available, one of his senior management team. The reason for this is that you must be briefed regarding forthcoming developments in the hospital, be they new buildings, new clinics or a new approach to the delivery of medical care to the local community. You can gain a great deal of information by talking to top-level managers, and much of this information may not be known to the consultant staff who will be interviewing you. Having learned high quality and up-to-date information from the managers, you can sound highly impressive by discussing the way in which the hospital is going to evolve during the next few years and how you feel that you, as a junior doctor, specialist registrar or as a consultant, will contribute to 'this blossoming service'. Additionally, and particularly if you are applying for a post at relatively senior level, make sure that you meet one or two consultants from related specialties. So, for example, if you are going for a post in cardiology then ensure you meet some of the cardiac surgeons. If you were applying for a post as a transplant surgeon, then the medical nephrologists and hepatologists would almost certainly be flattered if you took the trouble to meet them prior to the interview. Do not underestimate the extent to which potential candidates are discussed over the table in the consultants' dining room, and if your name is mentioned favourably here, it can work wonders in the final reckoning.

If you are struggling to meet the relevant consultants and senior members of the hospital management team, then consider trying to track down the president of the junior doctors' mess. The mess president is very likely to be able to give you up-to-date information regarding what is good and what is bad about the hospital. He may be able to introduce you to foundation year doctors and specialist registrars in the department to which you are applying, all of whom could be very useful sources of information, and conversation with them could result in you appearing far better informed than your competitors in the eventual job interview.

HOW TO CHOOSE A WINNING REFEREE

Selection of referees is not as immediately simple as it might seem. Your priority must be to choose people who will say nice things about you. However, some referees are all too willing to give a reference that is remarkably mediocre and does not make you stand out in comparison with the competition. Therefore, you need to go and speak to your potential referees and be prepared to ask them outright if they would be willing to write a *good* reference for you. This may seem to be a rather pushy approach, but there is no doubt that some senior medical staff will willingly agree to be a referee and then write rather uninspired comments which look bad when it comes to the interview. Short, matter-of-fact references never help anybody. So feel free to ask your potential referee if they would be willing to write a detailed reference, outlining your good points and explaining the reasons why you would be very suitable for the post which you are proposing to apply for. Also, do not hesitate to obtain a larger number of referees than was specifically requested in the job description and advertisement. We advise people that if the request is for two references then the names of three referees should be given. If the request is for three referees then four names should be offered. The main reason for this is that hospital personnel departments frequently request references at very short notice and sometimes referees are away or abroad. Failure to produce a reference is a total catastrophe. You must, therefore, offer the names of 'stand-by' referees. Moreover, many personnel departments will simply seek a reference from all of the names given as potential referees without thinking how many they originally specified. If an interview panel is deluged with a large number of strongly worded, glowing references speaking about you in the highest possible terms, then this can do nothing but good.

POINTS FOR REFLECTION

- Where and when will your chosen job be advertised?
- Are you familiar with the department you are applying to work in? If not, have you made plans to visit and meet some 'key players'?
- Who are you going to ask to act as your referees?

THE PERSON SPECIFICATION FORM – IGNORE IT AT YOUR PERIL!

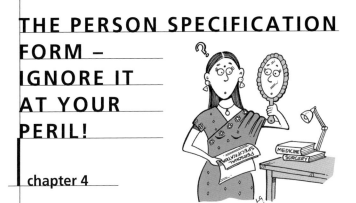

chapter 4

The person specification form is the most important document of the application process. Ignore it at your peril as it acts as the blueprint against which your online application form and interview responses will ultimately be scored. Person specifications for all specialties are available on the MMC websites. Take time to look through these, several months before the application process begins.

A number of standard, generic themes run through all of the person specifications (Table 4.1). Recognising this allows you to anticipate the type of question you may be asked during the application process and time to prepare your own individualised responses. Read the form carefully, since if you do not fulfil all of the essential entry criteria your application will fail immediately. The document indicates very clearly which criteria will be assessed in the online application process and which will be assessed at interview.

Getting that Medical Job: Secrets for Success, 3rd edition. © Colin J. Mumford and Suvankar Pal. Published 2011 by Blackwell Publishing Ltd.

Table 4.1 Example person specification form for application to a specialty training programme with some tips on how to succeed

Essential entry criteria

		When evaluated
Qualifications	MBBS or equivalent medical qualification **ST3 or above:** Success in Royal College examinations	**Application form**
Eligibility	Eligible for full registration with the GMC at time of appointment and hold a current licence to practice	**Application form** Interview/selection centre
	For ST1 level entry:	
	Evidence of achievement of foundation competencies	
	For ST3 level entry:	
	Evidence of achievement of **ST1 and ST2 competences** supported by evidence from workplace-based assessments of clinical performance (DOPS, Mini-CEX, CBD, ACAT) and Multi-source Feedback or equivalent *Tip: Keep your portfolio up to date!*	
	Competencies as outlined by GMC Good Medical Practice Guide	
	Good clinical care, maintaining good medical practice	
	Good relationships and communication with patients	
	Good working relationships with colleagues	
	Good teaching and training	
	Professional behaviour and probity	
	Delivery of good acute clinical care	
	Tip: Read the GMC Good Medical Practice Guide before you embark on the application process	

Table 4.1 (*Continued*)

Essential entry criteria		When evaluated
	http://www.gmc-uk.org/guidance/	
	Eligibility to work in the United Kingdom	
Fitness To Practise	Is up-to-date and fit to practise safely	**Application form** References
Language Skills	All applicants to have demonstrable skills in written and spoken English adequate to enable effective communication about medical topics with patients and colleagues	**Application form** Interview/selection centre
Health	Meets professional health requirements (in line with GMC standards/Good Medical Practice)	**Application form** Pre-employment health screening
Career Progression	Ability to provide a complete employment history with no unexplained career gaps	**Application form**
	• Evidence that career progression is consistent with personal circumstances • Evidence that present achievement and performance is commensurate with totality of period of training	
	Tip: Be prepared to explain gaps in your training	
Application Completion	ALL sections of application form completed FULLY according to written guidelines	**Application form**

Table 4.1 (*Continued*)

Further selection criteria – specific to specialty

	Essential	Desirable	When evaluated
Qualifications	As above	Intercalated BSc or equivalent (some offer marks depending on degree classification) **ST3 and above**: Royal College Examinations Higher degree – MSc/MD/PhD	**Application form** Interview/selection centre
Clinical experience	Evidence of competence in management of common emergencies and inpatients through continuous work-based assessments or equivalent	**ST3 and above**: Experience of relevant specialties at ST1/2 Evidence of training in critical care specialties	**Application form** Interview/selection centre References
Clinical skills	**Clinical knowledge and expertise**: Appropriate knowledge base and capacity to apply sound clinical judgement to problems	Attendance at relevant courses, e. g. ATLS, EPLS, APLS or equivalent	**Application form** Interview/selection centre References

Table 4.1 (*Continued*)

	Essential	Desirable	When evaluated
	Able to prioritise clinical need and aware of the basics of managing acutely ill patients		
	Demonstrate current ALS certification or equivalent		
Academic/ research skills	**Research skills**: Demonstrates understanding of the importance of audit and research, including awareness of ethical issues	Evidence of relevant academic and research achievements, e. g. degrees, prizes, awards, distinctions, grants, publications, presentations, other achievements	**Application form** Interview/selection centre
	Evidence of active participation in audit	Evidence of a portfolio of audit projects including where the audit loop has been closed	
	Teaching: Evidence of teaching experience and/or training in teaching	Evidence of clinical governance training or equivalent	
		Evidence of involvement in teaching students and/or other professionals	
		IT skills: Demonstrates information technology skills	

Table 4.1 (*Continued*)

	Essential	Desirable	When evaluated
Personal skills	*Tip: You must be able to demonstrate these personal skills giving examples unique to your own experience. Remember that examples may refer to clinical and non-clinical experiences.*	Evidence from multisource feedback or other work-based assessments of good multidisciplinary team working.	**Application form** Interview / Selection centre References
	Vigilance and situational awareness:		
	Capacity to be alert to dangers or problems, particularly in relation to clinical governance		
	Capacity to monitor developing situations and anticipate issues		
	Coping with pressure:		
	Capacity to operate under pressure		
	Demonstrates initiative and resilience to cope with setbacks and adapt to rapidly changing circumstances		
	Awareness of own limitations and when to ask for help		
	Managing others and team involvement:		
	Capacity to work cooperatively with others and work effectively in multiprofessional teams		

Table 4.1 (*Continued*)

	Essential	Desirable	When evaluated
	Capacity to demonstrate leadership when appropriate, e. g. supervising junior staff		
	Problem solving and decision-making:		
	Capacity to use logical/lateral thinking to solve problems and make decisions		
	Empathy and sensitivity:		
	Capacity to take in others' perspectives and treat others with understanding; sees patients as people		
	Communication skills:		
	Demonstrates clarity in written/spoken communication and capacity to adapt language as appropriate to the situation		
	Able to build rapport, listen, persuade and negotiate		
	Organisation and planning:		
	Capacity to organise oneself, prioritise own work and organise ward rounds		
	Demonstrates punctuality, preparation and self-discipline		
	Basic IT skills		
Probity	**Professional integrity and respect for others:**		**Application form**
	Capacity to take responsibility for own actions and demonstrate a non-judgemental approach towards others		Interview/selection centre
	Displays honesty, integrity, awareness of confidentiality and ethical issues		References

Table 4.1 (*Continued*)

	Essential	Desirable	When evaluated
Commitment To Specialty	**Learning and personal development:** Demonstrates interest and realistic insight into acute medicine Demonstrates self-awareness and ability to accept feedback Evidence of self-reflective practice Evidence of attendance at organised teaching and training programmes during training programmes	Extracurricular activities/ achievements relevant to specialty	**Application form** Interview/election centre References

Broadly speaking, the person specification is divided into sections including:

ESSENTIAL ENTRY CRITERIA

- Qualifications
- Minimal clinical experience related to level of application
- Fitness to practice
- Language skills
- Health
- Adequate career progression
- Completed application form!

SPECIALTY SPECIFIC SELECTION CRITERIA

- Qualifications
- Clinical experience
- Clinical skills
- Academic/Research skills
- Personal skills
- Probity
- Commitment to specialty

Remember to refer back regularly to the person specification form when completing online answers to ensure you are fulfilling all of the essential criteria and as many of the desirable criteria as possible. In the build up to your interview, practise giving responses to interview questions and ask friends and colleagues to score your answers using the person specification criteria as the reference marking scheme.

POINTS FOR REFLECTION

- Have you reviewed the person specification form for the job for which you are applying?
- Do you fulfil all the essential criteria?
- Do you meet all the desirable criteria? If not, what can you do between now and the application period to improve your chances of being shortlisted?

THE CURRICULUM VITAE: DO YOU STILL NEED ONE, AND HOW TO GET IT RIGHT

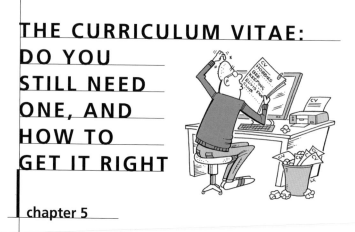

chapter 5

DO YOU STILL NEED A CV?

The adoption of the online application process for many posts has caused trainees to question whether they still need to prepare a decent curriculum vitae (CV), usually called a 'résumé' by our colleagues in North America. Understandably, candidates who are faced with computer screens requesting information about current posts, previous positions, special things that they have achieved in the past, and interrogation about 'challenging experiences' and 'situations in which you felt uncomfortable' feel that there is no place for the old-fashioned document made up of a fistful of A4 pages. But the CV remains vital for an appointment at consultant level, and can also be enormously helpful when applying for more junior posts. It can be used to supplement a top quality internet-based application, and is useful to leave behind when making early (or

Getting that Medical Job: Secrets for Success, 3rd edition. © Colin J. Mumford and Suvankar Pal. Published 2011 by Blackwell Publishing Ltd.

last-minute) visits to potential new workplaces and when meeting possible new senior colleagues. There is nothing to stop you taking paper copies of your CV into an interview, even when everything that has been done previously in the application process has been web-based. So *all* candidates should still have a CV 'up their sleeve', and that document should be perfect.

PRESENTATION

Entire books are devoted to the right and wrong ways to present a CV. Many formats are acceptable, but the document that is presented must be pristine. It must be laser printed and laid out in a simple, readily accessible format. Make sure that the typing is broadly spaced, and that dates describing the time spent in previous posts are clearly laid out. Modern interview panels, especially for senior appointments, take great pains to ensure that candidates have done the appropriate amount of general professional training and specialist training prior to appointment, and this is usually done right at the start of the interview. Watching a member of the interview panel struggling to piece together information from a poorly set out CV is desperately embarrassing and generally means rapid failure for the guilty candidate.

PROFESSIONAL COMPANY?

The back pages of the *British Medical Journal* are now awash with advertisements for professional companies who offer to present your CV in a 'better format'. Unless you are absolutely confident that you have achieved the optimal presentation of your own CV, it may be worth employing the services of one of these companies. Provided you can afford it, send off your CV, pay the money, and see what they produce. You may be pleasantly surprised to see how much improvement these companies can make, and if you are impressed with the new look of your own CV then it is very probable that those individuals constructing the shortlist or making the final appointment will also be impressed.

ORDER OF JOBS

Most medical CVs are set out in a certain order, usually starting with personal details, education, medical degrees, medical diplomas and higher qualifications, as well as noting registration with the General Medical Council (provisional, full or limited) and membership of a defence organisation. The CV should then describe your present and previous occupations. Unfortunately, this latter point is not as immediately simple as it sounds. Senior medical staff, and probably medical personnel departments as well, seem to be divided into two camps: those that like to see your present job first, with previous posts presented in reverse chronological order, and those that prefer your CV to read like a story book with your junior house officer (or FY1) posts first, then senior house officer (or FY2) posts, registrar posts and so on. Passions run surprisingly high in this area, but there is very little that you, as the interview candidate, can do in terms of 'mind reading' regarding what the shortlisters will prefer. Our own opinion is that interview panels are generally most interested in what you're doing *now*, and rather less interested in what you have done in the past. Therefore,we would advise going for the reverse chronological order approach, but be aware that it may slightly irritate some people.

Remember to make your present appointment sound as attractive as possible. For example, you may think that you are simply 'specialist registrar in general medicine', but if you think carefully you might find that you are also an honorary lecturer in medicine of the relevant university, or at least a clinical tutor to one or more medical students. All of these facets of your present post should be clearly stated.

GAPS ON THE CV

When describing previous appointments, make sure, above all, that the dates between which each post was held are clearly set out. List the names of the consultants for whom you worked. If you have performed locum posts try to fit these in, in chronological order. In recent years, the length of postgraduate training between foundation year and consultant posts in medical specialties has tended to shorten, and it has become increasingly important that interview panels are completely certain that all the training requirements needed for appointment to a given post have been completed.

Unexpected gaps in the sequence of jobs in your CV will lead to confusion, and this is to be avoided during the interview. If there are any periods of time in your CV which are unaccounted for, then be certain that you have included a comment to explain what you did during that vacant period. Even if this was time spent in an activity which you feel would not enhance your medical career then you should still include an explanation. Mysterious blanks trouble interview panels. Some candidates nowadays consider presenting their CV with a sort of 'time-line' down the right-hand margin of the pages which detail their career progress, so making it easier for interview panels to follow exactly what they have done since qualification, and this is a good idea.

OTHER CONTENT

Once you have dealt with present and previous posts in your CV then most interview panels like to see short sections describing your experience in your chosen specialty, teaching experience, management experience and, of course, a detailed description of research and audit work that you have done. You may wish to include a section listing courses and conferences attended. If you are applying for a relatively senior post it is likely that you will have a number of publications and these should be presented in detail. Traditionally, published work is presented in the following order:

- Books
- Chapters in books
- Refereed papers
- Review articles
- Invited editorials
- Published abstracts of communications to learned societies
- Published correspondence
- Poster presentations
- Finally, any non-medical publications which you may have.

You should conclude your CV by incorporating a section on your career development aims, other relevant information, for example languages spoken and information technology skills, and a short section on your interests and hobbies. The final page should be a list of your referees.

'DANGEROUS' CV CONTENT

It is difficult to imagine that anything you include in your CV might unintentionally threaten your success in the interview. Nevertheless, it is possible to put things in your CV which might be better left out. Most frequently, this problem arises with your list of 'hobbies and interests'. We would urge great caution before going into any detail regarding your membership of political organisations, and also beware of listing your enthusiasm for other groups which may seem innocuous to you, but which might not find favour with some of the more conservative members of the interview panel.

Everyone would agree that it would be foolhardy to list membership of an extremist or violent political organisation in your CV, but one of the authors was once alarmed to hear that a member of an interview panel drew the attention of a candidate to the fact that he had placed 'member of Amnesty International' under his interests. The interviewee was then asked whether he thought that this was a 'suitable thing' to place in a medical CV. Most of us would be horrified that such a question was asked, and the candidate apparently handled the issue extremely well, but this illustrates the fact that some thought is required regarding the presentation of your interests, since you can never account for unpredictable political leanings of the panel.

CONTACT DETAILS FOR YOUR REFEREES

The final page of your CV will be a list of your referees.We have already suggested that you should offer the names of one or two more referees than were originally asked for in the job specification. You *must* give comprehensive contact details for all your referees, since human resources departments have a very bad habit of seeking references for candidates only on the morning of the interview, or possibly no more than one or two days beforehand. Very frequently, these departments leave it too late to approach the relevant referee by mail, and they then cannot track them down by phone, so contact by fax or e-mail can sometimes save the day.

So, remember to make sure that you give the correct phone numbers (both direct line and hospital switchboard), the fax number and also the e-mail address for each of your referees, since details about you might well be requested at very short notice.

One final observation is required regarding your CV: do not take it for granted that the main 'selling point' which features in your CV will automatically come out during the interview. It may well be overlooked, and therefore it is up to you to make certain that the interview panel takes notice. Do not assume that they've read something; you need to say it!

POINTS FOR REFLECTION

- When did you last update your CV?
- Have you showcased all your achievements?
- Have you accounted for career gaps?
- Have your referees reviewed your CV and provided accurate contact details?

HOW TO DEAL WITH THE ONLINE APPLICATION FORM FOR FOUNDATION YEAR APPLICATIONS – 'RADIATING EXCELLENCE IN 250 WORDS OR LESS'

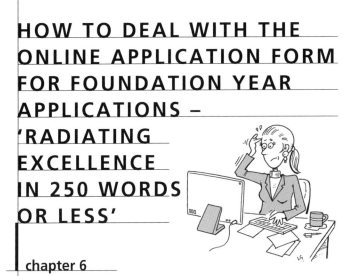

chapter 6

BACKGROUND

Foundation training is made up of a 2-year general educational programme which begins after completion of medical school. Most programmes involve a rotation through 4-month placements with exposure to different specialities, perhaps including general medicine, surgery, paediatrics, obstetrics and gynaecology, and general practice. Full registration with the General Medical Council occurs after completion of the FY1 year, which may be considered an extension of the traditional 5-year undergraduate programme.

Following the immense changes imposed by the 'modernising medical careers' debacle, Foundation Year applications

Getting that Medical Job: Secrets for Success, 3rd edition. © Colin J. Mumford and Suvankar Pal. Published 2011 by Blackwell Publishing Ltd.

are now made only once per year, and take place across the whole of the United Kingdom by means of an online application process. At the time of writing this book, there was a possibility that this nation-wide approach would change back to a rather more user-friendly local or regional application process, and this may be the case by the time you are reading this. Remarkably, there are currently no interviews for these junior posts. Instead, candidates are simply ranked according to a combination of scores based on medical school performance and their application form responses. At present, undergraduate performance is established by quartile ranking in medical school examinations and contributes 40% of the overall ranking mark. The same scoring system applies across all medical schools in the United Kingdom and applicants do not score any extra points for graduating from universities traditionally perceived as being more 'prestigious' such as Oxford or Cambridge. 60% of the overall ranking mark is based on assessment of responses to an online application form. This is one of the frustrating and disliked aspects of the online process, since consistently excelling for 5 or 6 years at medical school offers no guarantee of success in securing the desired FY job and so considerable time and effort needs to be devoted to getting the online form right!

WHAT MAKES A CANDIDATE STAND OUT?

It may at first seem as though there is very little to separate candidates applying for Foundation Year posts in terms of experience and qualifications. After all, undergraduate curricula are broadly very similar. But candidates who reflect more deeply on their unique attributes and experiences tend to score much better in their online responses. In particular, think about how your achievements in any of the following areas make you stand out:
• Undergraduate prizes and awards
• Intercalated BSc/BMedSci/PhD dissertations and research projects

- Overseas elective experience
- Special study module projects
- Contribution to medical school life (sporting, musical, theatrical and so on)
- Voluntary work (medical or otherwise)
- Paid employment during your study (phlebotomy, medical secretary, even work in the student bar!)
- Work experience before entering medicine

EXAMPLE QUESTIONS

Question 1

Give two examples of specific learning needs that you identified as part of your undergraduate medical training. Compare and contrast your approaches to addressing these differing needs. How will you use these experiences to develop your competence and performance as a foundation doctor?

A good answer

One learning need I identified during training was the skill of history taking. To address this, I observed clinicians in practice and consulted clinical texts. Whilst this provided me with a framework for history taking, I found the most benefit came from directly practising, at first with peers, and then by speaking to as many patients as possible during clinical attachments. Approaching patients at their most vulnerable was not easy at first, but the overwhelming majority were extremely supportive and I have succeeded in developing a confident bedside manner, putting patients at ease and formulating differential diagnoses. By guiding younger colleagues on the process of history taking, I have been able to reflect on my own technique and strive continually to improve my communication skills and diagnostic formulations during my career.

Developing competence in venepuncture was another learning need addressed. Although I initially studied protocols, as with history

*taking, this skill required a direct practical approach and I sought op-
portunities to practise the technique, initially on model arms in facili-
tated clinical skills centres, and then on the wards under senior supervision whilst always appreciating my limitations. When I felt appropriately confident, I performed the procedure unsupervised as I assisted
in clinics and I am now able to teach other students. As a foundation
doctor, I will continue to address learning needs by acquiring information, practising, receiving constructive criticism and reflecting on
my achievements. I will apply such an approach to my everyday work,
confidently and efficiently carrying out the skills I have attained whilst
learning new ones, always seeking ways to improve in order to further
develop my competence and performance as a practitioner.*

Question 2

Compare and contrast the care that you have observed for two
patients with the same diagnosis and similar clinical problems.
Describe the care, and the extent to which it took into account
the individual needs of the patients. What have you learned
from these observations and how will you apply this learning
to your future clinical practice?

A good answer

*Two young patients with schizophrenia, one whom I saw in Fiji on my
elective period, and one in the UK, were experiencing distressing hal-
lucinations and delusions, symptoms which were also interfering with
their personal relationships. The Fijian patient had been placed in a
general medical ward due to lack of sufficient psychiatric services, with
the intention of relocating her to an elderly people's home, whereas the
UK patient was receiving long-term care in a specialist rehabilitation
centre. Both patients were receiving similar drug therapy. The UK specialist services took the time to listen to their patient, considering their
psychological needs and addressing the patient's requirements without presuming that such needs would be the same every day. The care
provided was therefore always contextual and necessary. The social*

circumstances of the UK patient were appreciated, with relatives and friends acknowledged in the care plan where possible, whereas in contrast, the Fijian patient had the same management plan throughout her hospital stay and her personal relationships were not regarded with such importance.

These encounters taught me how patients can have the same diagnosis but in order to provide optimal care their entire biopsychosocial situation must be considered rather than drug therapy alone. The Westernised world seems better at acknowledging and providing the facilities to address all three of these aspects, and consequently the care I observed for the UK patient seemed far more impressive and patient-sensitive. Such observations have shown me the importance of individualised patient-centred care, an approach I aim to adopt as a future practitioner.

Question 3

Describe one example of a clinical situation where you demonstrated or observed appropriate professional behaviour despite difficult circumstances. How will you apply what you have learned to your future practice?

A good answer

The first cardiac arrest I witnessed occurred in a small, limited resource, accident and emergency department. Despite being apprehensive, I knew I had the skills to help and so took the initiative to assist in the resuscitation. In spite of the difficult circumstances, teamwork prevailed and I participated in chest compressions and ventilation. The patient died and the distressed family was informed in an admirably professional manner, the doctor honestly acknowledging the limitations of the department and clearly and respectfully explaining the events leading to the death.

This experience taught me that in medicine, there will be inevitably difficult circumstances and although I may lack confidence, it is better to take the initiative and provide assistance whilst maintaining integrity and probity. I will regard future encounters as learning experiences, whilst simultaneously providing essential patient care and will endeavour to be honest and respectful when faced with difficult situations.

Question 4

Describe one example, not necessarily clinical, that has increased your understanding of team working. Describe your role and how you contributed to the team. What have you learned and how will you apply this to working with colleagues as a foundation doctor?

A good answer

My understanding of teamwork improved during a trip to Bosnia with Students for Children International Projects charity. As part of a small group of students, I visited separate childcare organisations and helped in deciding which was the most in need of volunteers. After passionate debate, we eventually agreed on a particular orphanage; though abandoning other projects caused many tears. We began sourcing potential sponsors and devising fundraisers. I contributed by leading publicity, which involved organising events, advertising and recruiting students. This project has taught me much about respecting the opinions of others and accepting team decisions. I have learnt that each person brings individual skills to a group and the result is often greater than the sum of the parts. I will apply this as a foundation doctor by attempting to value all opinions and by respecting delegation by the team leader, as understanding the components of teamwork will be essential for good patient care.

Question 5

Describe a situation, not necessarily clinical, where you personally felt challenged and under pressure. Describe how you responded. What did you learn from this experience and how will this benefit you as a foundation doctor?

A good answer

During my obstetrics attachment, a patient presented with a deep vein thrombosis (DVT). On admission, it was discovered she had right-sided renal carcinoma and an ovarian tumour. Her prognosis was poor. She didn't understand what the doctors had told her and asked me to explain. It was very challenging to communicate such bad news; more so, as she was simply expecting treatment for a DVT. First, I established how much she knew and what she wished to be explained. I then talked her through her diagnosis, explaining as clearly as I could. She didn't wish to know her prognosis so it wasn't discussed. She thanked me for talking to her as she said nobody else had. I indicated I would mention it to one of the doctors in case she had further questions. This difficult experience taught me how important it is to listen to the patient and to communicate simply, clearly, and with empathy.

Question 6

Describe one of your non-academic achievements. Explain clearly why this was an achievement for you. What did you learn from this achievement and how will this influence your approach to patient care?

A good answer

For my elective, I undertook 8 weeks of paediatrics in a French hospital. I studied French at school but had no French medical vocabulary. To prepare, I ordered several French textbooks, and during my paediatrics attachment I reviewed each day's teachings and then studied the same topics in French. On completion of my attachment, I had also completed the entire paediatrics syllabus in French. In France, I worked in A&E clerking in patients, and often presented patients on ward rounds. It was a significant achievement to work in a different language and environment, and to have taught myself enough French medical vocabulary to do so successfully. To achieve this required self-discipline and a clear focus. I planned ahead, and committed to the extra work required. Maintaining this focus on objectives, and thorough, advance preparation to achieve them, will ensure I provide patients with the highest levels of care and attention.

GENERAL TIPS

The strongest answers:
- reflect on individual experiences giving more personalised responses;
- are clear and concise in their description (every word must count!); and
- reflect on how learning experiences will be of benefit during foundation training.

POINT FOR REFLECTION

- What experiences and achievements (academic, extracurricular, overseas elective, special study modules) were unique to you as an undergraduate?

HOW TO DEAL WITH THE ONLINE APPLICATION FORM FOR SPECIALTY TRAINEE (ST) APPLICATIONS

chapter 7

BACKGROUND

The time available to complete and submit online application forms is only a matter of weeks. It is therefore important to anticipate questions and have responses ready for those points which will undoubtedly feature on the form. As with Foundation Year application responses, the best applications to Specialty Trainee (ST) posts are those which reflect on personal attributes and achievements. At this stage questions almost invariably focus on the following areas:

1 Clinical experience
2 Personal achievements and qualities
3 Audit, presentations and publications
4 Teaching experience
5 Leadership skills
6 Ethical awareness
7 Commitment to specialty

Getting that Medical Job: Secrets for Success, 3rd edition. © Colin J. Mumford and Suvankar Pal. Published 2011 by Blackwell Publishing Ltd.

Remember that online responses will be restricted by specific word counts so answers should be concise and there is no room for waffle. Seek feedback on your responses from people who know you well. Don't be afraid to ask the advice of friends, applicants from recent years and senior colleagues in your chosen specialty. Be prepared to accept criticism and adapt your answers accordingly. Research all resources available early on in the application process including deanery, Royal College, and national recruitment programme websites.

EXAMPLE QUESTIONS AND ANSWERS

1. CLINICAL EXPERIENCE

Please highlight below the competences you have achieved that are particularly relevant to this application

Remember to include specific clinical experience related to the specialty, competency in relevant clinical procedures, level of involvement in acute take, and outpatient and inpatient work. Also refer to relevant clinical courses attended and any research or audit you have participated in.

Example answer: ST1 application for core medical training (CMT)

As an FY1, I worked in the medical admitting unit of a district general hospital. I gained experience in assessment and management of patients with unselected medical presentations. I am currently building on this experience over 4 months in a more senior role in the admissions unit of a busy regional teaching hospital. In addition to clerking and initiating management, I am responsible for maintaining an overview of patients and providing support for FY1s. I am aware of limitations as a junior doctor and am consolidating skills in how and when to make appropriate referrals to seniors and other specialties. I have worked in a regional neurosciences centre, regularly assessing patients with acute neurological presentations. As an FY1 I rotated through surgical HDU, where I learnt to assess confidently acutely unwell patients, initiate treatment and seek help where appropriate. I have been part of the arrest team in all previous attachments and have strengthened this experience with an ALS course. I am competent in the FY curriculum procedures. In addition, I have performed numerous lumbar punctures, ascitic taps and external ventricular drains independently, pleural taps under supervision, and have placed a chest and an ascitic drain.

Example answer: ST1 application for basic surgical training (BST)

Clinical experience: Four months as an FY1 in General Surgery, 4 months as an FY1 in Thoracic Surgery and 4 months as an FY2 managing neurosurgical patients out of hours on the ward and in HDU. Currently assessing gynaecology patients pre- and post-operatively and gaining experience in obstetric and gynaecology theatres. Six-week medical student elective in neurosurgery was primarily spent assisting in theatre. These experiences have exposed me extensively to the pre-operative assessment and investigation of surgical patients, their surgical management and post-operative management on wards and in HDU. As such, they have developed my surgical knowledge, practical skills and clinical experience in the assessment, management and investigation of surgical patients. They have given me the capacity to operate effectively under pressure, to prioritise clinical need and have further developed my problem-solving skills. My general medical FY1 job also developed my medical knowledge and ability to manage common medical conditions, important clinical experience for the management of surgical patients.

***Surgical experience**: As a medical student, I took the opportunity to go to theatre as much as possible. My 6-week medical elective was spent mainly assisting in neurosurgical theatres. In each of my Foundation jobs I have taken the opportunity to go to theatre and* *assist where possible, as reflected by entries into my surgical logbook. I have also taken the opportunity to work with anaesthetists, to gain experience of intubation, line insertion, intra-operative monitoring of patients and their management on HDU and ITU. Where possible I have assisted with, and performed, ward-based procedures such as aspiration of ascitic fluid and insertion of ascitic drains, insertion of chest drains, lumbar punctures and minor suturing of wounds, as documented in my surgical logbook and e-portfolio. Attended and passed the Royal College of Surgeons Basic Surgical Skills Course.*

*   **Courses and examinations:** I have continued to gain surgical knowledge throughout foundation year training by study for MRCS Part A and attendance of ALS, ATLS, Basic Surgical Skills and CCRISP courses. I am currently preparing for MRCS Part B.*

*   **Research experience:** I have been involved in a variety of research projects throughout medical school and foundation years, from audit to literature review to case reports.*

2. PERSONAL ATTRIBUTES AND QUALITIES

Describe, with examples, how your personal skills and attributes make you suitable for a career in this specialty

Answers to this type of question should be relevant to the post being applied for. Marks are specifically allocated to qualities identified in the person specification form as desirable, including communication skills, empathy and sensitivity, conceptual thinking, problem solving, managing others, teamwork, coping with pressure, dealing with ambiguity, organisation and planning, vigilance and situational awareness. Remember that personal achievements and qualities include non-medical activities you have participated in.

Example answer for ST1 post in psychiatry

Study for a BA (Hons) in music at York University allowed me to refine my critical thinking skills and ability to write concisely on abstract subjects. Participation in orchestras and ensembles, private music teaching, and voluntary work leading students in music sessions at special schools in York demanded sensitive team-working and leadership abilities. Between my music degree and starting medical school, employment supporting adults with learning disabilities for 1 year and auxiliary nursing for 6 months required competent and adaptable communication skills which have been invaluable since. During medical school, I furthered my non-judgemental supportive communication skills as a Samaritans volunteer.

Maturity and experience has equipped me with effective ways of dealing with pressure, and this has been useful during busy foundation jobs in colorectal surgery, medicine of the elderly, and in medicine at the Victoria Hospital in Kirkcaldy. Proficient time management and planning allowed me to undertake time-consuming audit projects as a medical FY1 in Kirkcaldy and as a psychiatry FY2 at the Royal Edinburgh Hospital. Extracurricular activities including climbing, music, and recently skiing, replenish my energy so that I continue to enjoy working under pressure. I am enjoying the greater responsibility of FY2. In particular, work at the Alcohol Problems Service at the Royal Edinburgh Hospital gave me confidence in assessing and managing alcohol and drug problems in inpatient and outpatient settings. Out-of-hours shifts covering all psychiatry wards required me to assess acutely unwell patients, make sensible assessments of risk to myself and others, and make short-term plans for dealing with risk. I am drawn to uncertainty within medicine, and in my current neurology post am working on a research project on functional weakness: an area where tests and treatments often fall short. I look forward to dealing with the uncertainties that a career in psychiatry will afford.

Example answer for CMT application

As a member of my college and Cambridge medical school boat clubs in 2002-2006, I regularly competed successfully within the university. I competed in an international race in Nantes in 2004 for crews from universities around Europe. As I gained experience, I took on a more senior role on the committee as 2nd boat captain in 2003–04. This has allowed me to develop my organisational skills and given me valuable experience of performing within and leading a team. I enjoy running and completed two half-marathons in 2006 and 2009 finishing within the top 500 in my category, fitting training around my work commitments and raising over a thousand pounds for Médecins Sans Frontières. This taught me a lot about hard work and determination. I completed my level 2 dinghy sailing course in 2009, where I had to learn to sail as part of a small team, and to monitor the many other boats close by and anticipate any changes occurring on the water. White-water rafting the Grand Canyon in 2009 was a further experience of working as a close-knit team. I enjoy learning languages and am bilingual in German, have a GCSE equivalent in Italian, and have a certificate in basic French.

3. AUDIT, PRESENTATIONS AND PUBLICATIONS

Please detail your involvement in audit and research. What publications and presentations have you made?

For this answer, specify to what extent you initiated any research or audit work. Detail your involvement and highlight specific methodologies you have gained experience in. For audits, highlight if the 'audit loop' has been completed and how practice has changed as a result of your findings. Provide details of meetings you have presented at and publication formats and journal articles you may have authored.

Example answer for CMT post

Audit

'Smoking cessation support in aneurysmal subarachnoid haemorrhage'. Edinburgh, Aug.—Nov. 2008.

I initiated and designed this clinical audit. I collated information from 80 patients presenting with aneurysmal subarachnoid haemorrhage to the regional neurosciences unit throughout 2008. I analysed the results myself and presented the audit at the Scottish Association of Neurological Sciences conference in November 2008. I hope to continue work to implement recommended changes to current clinical practice in this area.

Manuscript in preparation for Journal of smoking cessation (first author).

'Post-operative pain and side effects following intrathecal morphine'. Kirkcaldy, Dec. 2007–April 2008.

I identified this area for study after observing non-standardised practice in the use of intrathecal morphine in spinal anaesthetics for elective orthopaedic procedures. I designed a questionnaire to assess post-operative pain and side effects. I interviewed patients one to two days post-operatively and collated results. With some assistance in statistical analysis I completed and presented the audit at the departmental 'anaesthetics in-service' meeting. A standardised protocol has now been developed in Fife improving clinical practice and closing the audit loop.

'Effective Clinical Documentation'. Fife, March–May 2008.

I collated information within this ongoing audit designed to assess the level of confidentiality, effectiveness of documentation, and record keeping in the acute medical wards.

Research

First author publication in 'The Healing Hand' British Emmanuel Healthcare Journal. Volume 63, 2006. Elective Report 'Hawaiian Provision of Rural Healthcare Services'.

Second author 'Learning to take informed consent; an example of a professional skill influenced by the hidden curriculum'. Poster presented at The Association for the Study of Medical Education, Annual Scientific Meeting, Edinburgh 2003.

First author publication of health promotion calendar 'Healthcare Associated Infection' Western General Hospital, Edinburgh. Lothian Infection Control Team research project 2005–06.

Third author 'Accelerated long-term forgetting; a case study'. Department of Clinical Neurosciences, Western General Hospital, Edinburgh. In preparation for publication in 'Epilepsy'.

4. TEACHING

Please provide details of your involvement in teaching activities

Include examples of formal and informal teaching undertaken at undergraduate and postgraduate level. Include formats such as bedside teaching, seminars, lectures and teaching of specific skills such as practical procedures, history taking and communication skills. Include attendance at teaching courses and any qualifications in clinical education (e.g. Certificate, Diploma or MSc). Remember your teaching experience may not necessary all be medical in nature.

Example answer 1 for CMT post

In my final year, I was an associate clinical supervisor for a group of new clinical students, teaching them history and examination techniques in their first few weeks in a clinical setting. As part of finals revision, I prepared tutorials on areas of the curriculum. I currently deliver regular bedside and other clinical teaching to students attached to my team, and have given a tutorial on lumbar punctures to a small group of students, providing a handout of case studies from my neurology attachment. I am keen to become more involved in regular formal teaching and have recently signed up to give pharmacology tutorials for 3rd year students. Outside of medicine I have a considerable amount of teaching experience which has helped when teaching within medicine. I spent 3 months in Japan in 2003 teaching English at two language schools to varying ages and class sizes which required very different approaches. As a member of my college boat club from 2002–2005, I was regularly involved in coaching more junior members.

Example answer 2 for CMT post

During fifth year I organised 'peer mentor' tutorials for first year medical students. These formal sessions were available via the medical school website and covered issues ranging from stress with exams to coping with life at university. I acted as mentor to six students for one academic year and, following feedback to the medical school, a formal framework of similar tuition was implemented for subsequent years. During FY1 I designed and produced a clinical skills video for medical school applicants and students at Edinburgh University. This project included several open days at the 'clinical skills centre' where I demonstrated clinical skills. Such was the positive response from students and FY1s that a further set of clinical skills sessions were organised. During University I acted as student representative for my year group, this included a formal meeting each term with course organisers to discuss issues such as clinical placements, assessments and resources. During FY2 neurology placement I put this experience into practice. I organised the on-call rota for nine doctors covering three wards. I also initiated and coordinated a set of clinical teaching seminars with registrars and senior specialists. I have recently completed a health care skills course in 'clinical teaching'.

5. LEADERSHIP INVOLVEMENT

Please detail dates, type and level of any experience you have of leadership roles in either medical or non-medical fields

Include specific details of type of leadership roles, either medical or non-medical, for example working in a team or organisation. Include the level, for example local, national, school or university. Include work-related organisational activities such as rota co-ordinator or representative roles.

Example answer for CMT application

As an ambitious sportsperson I have stepped up to the challenge of captain for Edinburgh University 1st XI hockey team 2006–2007,

Scottish Universities and Ireland U21. As captain I took on a great deal of responsibility including organising National League fixtures, team selection and representation duties. Coinciding with my final year at medical school I became astute at time management, prioritisation and the appropriate delegation of tasks. On reflection this experience was invaluable for medical training. I learnt to integrate the strengths and personalities of the team members to achieve our maximum potential. I developed an approachable manner, and good communication throughout the team allowed individual perspectives to be respected. My national hockey captaincy was not without challenges and I learnt to cope with pressure and to anticipate problems. Balancing personal skills with clear team objectives and feedback I have seen many outcomes achieved. Motivation and commitment to my role as leader in sport has had a positive impact on my approach to teamwork within medicine. I have completed health care skills course in 'Teams and Leadership'. I believe leadership is one of my strengths and I hope to remain committed to efficient teamwork and confident leadership throughout my core medical training.

6. ETHICAL CONSIDERATIONS

Mistakes can and do happen in medical practice. Describe a specific example where the outcome of action you took in response to a clinical mistake/error (made by you or someone else) caused you to reassess how you subsequently dealt with similar situations. What action did you take at the time and how has your practice now changed?

ST3 application for neurology

I gained consent from a family for post mortem of a relative. They were extremely distressed by unexpected disfigurement of the body following the procedure and, in particular, that they were not warned of the potential for this. Action taken included convening a multidisciplinary meeting which culminated in acknowledgement of the family's complaint and a written apology from my supervising consultant. The family were invited to clinic and a further apology issued. A clinical incident form was completed and the matter recorded. In order to improve practice after this case I will take additional time, and if necessary seek expert advice, when seeking informed consent, particularly at times of distress. Following a meeting with the pathologist a standard operating procedure has been devised to improve delivery of informed consent for post mortem. The effectiveness of this intervention is to be monitored by auditing future similar complaints.

7. COMMITMENT TO SPECIALTY

Why are you motivated to pursue further training in this specialty? In what way are you able to demonstrate that your own skills and attributes are suitable for a higher career in this specialty?

ST3 application neurology

My specialty interest stems from pursuit of an intercalated BSc in neurosciences, neurology special study modules, an overseas elective, and an SHO position at the National Hospital for Neurology. My current post involves independent assessment of suspected CJD cases across the United Kingdom. I have repeatedly built rapport and demonstrated empathy and sensitivity towards patients with rapidly progressive neurological symptoms. Clinical assessments have contributed to problem solving and decision-making skills and in identifying patients' medical and psychosocial needs. My role involves working efficiently within a multiprofessional team and clear written and verbal communication with neurologists, patients and families. Concurrent pursuit of a laboratory-based thesis requires determination, initiative and an ability to cope with the demands of delivering a clinical service whilst undertaking research. This has strengthened skills of organisation, planning, prioritising work and performing under pressure. My ambition is to be a clinical neurologist with a special interest in neurodegenerative disease.

Personal statement in support of application to deanery

Example answer for CMT application

Throughout foundation training I have thrived on the diversity of clinical exposure within the medical specialties. I am a confident communicator with strengths in interpersonal skills and teamwork, with an aptitude for clinical skills. I have an eye for detail and the stamina and patience to untangle complicated medical problems. I understand the importance of continued education and research and the need to work directly with other specialties.

I enjoy the buzz and pace of hospital medicine. I hope to develop a good breadth of knowledge and skills that are essential to the provision of high quality health care whilst maintaining a patient-centred approach.

I will approach core medical training with enthusiasm, commitment and hard work.

This programme offers a well-designed and supported pathway of education, training and lifelong learning. I have enjoyed university and foundation training in this region, well supported and inspired by seniors.

The region also offers a great quality of life, with rich culture, friendly people and a wonderful range of sports and activities.

Example answer for psychiatry application

My unusual route into medicine via a music degree and support work with adults with learning disabilities gave me the benefits of a range of life experience and a keen social awareness. I was interested before medical school in mental illness and the effects it has on peoples' lives. At medical school, placements in old-age and forensic psychiatry and voluntary work with Samaritans increasingly drew me towards psychiatry as an intellectually challenging specialty where 'people' skills are key. As a foundation doctor in medical and surgical specialties I felt most rewarded by working with people with enduring health problems, with challenging patients and in difficult communication scenarios. As psychiatry FY2, I appreciated being able to spend more time with patients eliciting a detailed history and examining mental state, and enjoyed working as part of an effective multidisciplinary team. I relish the academic challenges offered by a career in psychiatry, and look forward to getting involved in research and study for higher postgraduate degrees. In particular, I am keen to benefit from the high-quality psychiatry training available in this region and to remain here in the longer term.

Example response for basic surgical training application

General Surgery is an exciting specialty with a wide variety of practical, clinical and intellectual challenges. There is a broad spread of clinical and operative work ranging from the management of benign and malignant disease to the acutely unwell patient. It encompasses a wide range of surgical techniques. Additionally, there are many opportunities to be involved in research and audit. My clinical, research and study experience, along with my personal attributes, have convinced me of the privilege and satisfaction of working in such a specialty. General surgical training in this region offers a broad and thorough training in General Surgery and the subspecialities. Training units provide a variety of district general services and tertiary referral exposure, giving the trainee a good volume and breadth of experience. The region has a long-standing international academic reputation leading, for example, in the fields of inflammation and transplant research. Finally, the quality of life here is undoubtedly exceptional with a wealth of physical pursuits and natural beauty.

POINTS FOR REFLECTION

Think about how you will structure your own application form answers in terms of:
• clinical experience;
• personal achievements and qualities;

- audit, presentations and publications;
- teaching experience;
- leadership skills;
- ethical awareness; and
- commitment to specialty.

THE INTERVIEW

chapter 8

WHERE, WHEN AND HOW?

The previous chapters have considered issues relating to the on-line application, how to deal with the forms used, and tips for specific types of answer. For junior-level appointments, completion of the online form may be the final event on which decisions are based, with no subsequent face-to-face interview. But for more senior appointments, there will inevitably be a formal interview, and it is now time to consider general aspects of that process.

If you have followed the instructions in the first part of this book, done the ground work, visited the right people, and excelled in your online application, then – if the appointment is going to be made based on interview, and not on the basis of the online process alone – with luck you will have made it onto the shortlist, and accordingly you will be invited to attend for interview. Like so many facets of getting on in a medical career, preparation for the interview needs to start even before you

Getting that Medical Job: Secrets for Success, 3rd edition. © Colin J. Mumford and Suvankar Pal. Published 2011 by Blackwell Publishing Ltd.

receive the letter inviting you to attend. Remember that you are not such an important candidate that the date, time or location of the interview will be changed just to suit you. Therefore, it is perfectly reasonable, when applying for a job, to ask the hospital personnel department if a date has already been set for the interview, and you should ensure that you are not on holiday or out of the country for another reason on the allotted date. Only under totally exceptional circumstances will you be able to persuade an interview panel to change the date of an interview, and this is only likely to happen for very senior appointments if you are clearly the front-running candidate.

The second vital issue, which sounds obvious but which is frequently a stumbling block for junior doctors, is the need to find out the exact location of the interview. This is not as simple as it may seem since frequently candidates assume that the interview will take place in the hospital at which they have applied for a job, whereas in fact the interview is held at the regional postgraduate centre, the Trust Board offices or the headquarters of the regional health authority. All these are traps for the unwary, and if this sort of elementary information is not sorted out at an early stage you will be rattled if you eventually do make it to the interview. There is nothing worse than turning up a few minutes late for an interview and having to apologise for being late because you went to the wrong venue. Under no circumstances whatsoever should you be late for the interview since to turn up late implies a degree of shoddy planning which will immediately alienate most senior doctors, who will think that if you are incapable of getting to an interview on time, then there is no chance at all that you will actually make it to their clinic, to their operating theatre session, or to their ward rounds on time.

It is perfectly reasonable to try to find out who will be interviewing you. Nowadays in Britain there tend not to be any interviews for FY1 and FY2 posts, since appointments are determined on the basis of the online application system alone, but they still occur in some places, and are often used for locum appointments. Candidates at junior level may be surprised to find a panel as small as two individuals. More frequently the panel is much larger than that, and for most specialist registrar appointments, and certainly for consultant grade appointments, the panel may be as big as 11 or 12 people. The reason for this is that most interview panels are now convened to a relatively set formula. There will be some of the consultants for whom you are going to be working, of course, but in addition, there will be representatives of the relevant university, somebody representing the regional postgraduate dean, and a member of the hospital management team. Bear in mind that this latter person may know very little about medicine and, indeed, may know surprisingly little about the day-to-day clinical workings of their own hospital. Increasingly, panels also now include a 'lay representative'. This individual is sometimes jokingly, and rather unfairly, referred to using the generic term, 'the vicar's wife'. They may ask some very unexpected questions, and it is worth being well prepared for the questions that may come from 'the vicar's wife', about which more later.

Note also that for specialist registrar and consultant appointments there will be another important individual who is the Royal College representative, previously referred to as the 'national panellist' for interviews in Scotland. This member of the panel has a slightly different remit, in that he is not there to assess who is best for the job, but to ensure that every candidate who attends the interview has done the required amount of previous training, for example general professional training before specialisation, and he also confirms to the chairman of the interview panel that you are 'suitable for appointment to the offered post'.

Remember also that although you may have spent many hours trying to 'bump into' the professor and head of department in the corridor outside his office, whilst he will almost certainly be on the panel, he will not usually be the chairman.

Rather the chairman of large interview panels tends now to be a consultant from a different specialty and sometimes from a different hospital. Alternatively, this person may be the medical director of the hospital in which you are applying to work. The chairman of the panel is there to ensure fair play and may not, in fact, have a vote in the final judgement as to who is appointed, but increasingly they do have a valid vote, so you need to win them over, just like the rest of the panel.

Knowing the individual members of the panel in advance can be enormously helpful in being successful in the medical job interview. Once you have heard that you are shortlisted, you should contact the relevant personnel department and ask if they are able to let you know the composition of the panel. Some hospitals are rather cagey about this, believing it is somehow 'unfair', but in general terms most personnel departments are willing to give you a list of names and job titles of the people comprising the panel. You should then find out exactly who they are, where they work and what they do. If you have not already met them on a previous visit then you may wish to make a further visit to ensure that your face is known to as many members of the panel as possible.

The interview itself is likely to be held in a large, relatively formal, room. Many hospitals have a 'boardroom' which they reserve almost exclusively for this purpose. In the same way that you must know exactly the geographical location of the interview building, you must also make absolutely sure that you can find your way to the correct room. Shrewd candidates also make careful note of the location of the nearest toilets.

WHAT TO WEAR

Clothing for an interview is largely a matter of personal choice but nevertheless the concept of 'power dressing' should be adhered to as far as possible. Whatever you select from your wardrobe, your goal must be to look entirely professional and

101% appropriate for the post for which you are applying. Most senior hospital physicians are relatively conservative people in the way they dress and they will expect you to do likewise. For men a dark suit with a pristine white shirt and contrasting tie is undoubtedly the most appropriate. Your shoes must be gleaming. Men should not wear any obvious jewellery simply because it runs the risk of alienating one or more members of the panel. You may, of course, wear a discreet tie clip and appropriate, unobtrusive cufflinks.

The choice of tie for men can be all important. Indeed, if you are forced into the 'uniform' of a dark suit and a white shirt, then the choice of a good tie is one of the few ways in which you can display some individuality. The tie should be of a pattern best described as 'classic'. For example, woven silk or plain silk with a simple pattern. Sometimes, relatively bright colours including red, orange and yellow can look quite striking and yet, at the same time, retain an air of great professionalism. We would urge caution against wearing any sort of club tie. Even if you happen to know that the head of department was in the same Royal Air Force squadron as your father, it is ill-advised to wear the appropriate club or regimental tie since you run the risk of being questioned about the tie and its significance. One of two things will then happen: either you will be able to answer in a very erudite manner impressing the former Group Captain on the interview panel, and this will alienate the other members; or, alternatively, you will not be able to answer the probing questions relating to the provenance of your tie and you will then look totally ridiculous. Club ties, therefore, are out.

Clothing for women is altogether more difficult and it is quite reasonable to ask for advice from senior female medical colleagues. You must, of course, aim to look smart, and the goal should be to look stylish and not 'frumpy' or 'tarty'. You should ensure that you choose clothing you feel comfortable in, which you can walk in and which you can sit down safely in! Either trousers or a skirt are acceptable as long as they are smart.

Whatever you choose, remember all the time that the guiding principle must be to appear totally professional. And remember to take a second pair of tights with you on the day; the pair that you are wearing when you leave home will inevitably be laddered when they get caught on the taxi door as you arrive at the interview!

One word on smell, and that is 'don't'. Excessive use of any cosmetics is to be avoided. Female candidates may, of course, risk a modest splash of perfume and apply make-up, but make-up should be done in a manner that gives a professional impression without looking garish. Small items of jewellery are also quite reasonable for women. In the same way that men should avoid jewellery, men should also avoid anything other than minimal application of aftershave. Most panels will object to what they perceive as a 'man wearing perfume'.

HOW TO SIT

It is possible to anticipate what will happen when you are called into the interview room. You will be sitting outside the room, usually with other candidates who will mostly not be engaging in conversation with you. When your name is called you need to stand up smartly and follow the invitation to enter the interview room. First impressions are all important and you need, as you go through the door, first to look professional, secondly to look interested in what is going on and thirdly—and above all—to start giving an immediate impression that you are the only suitable candidate for the job. One way to achieve this is to acknowledge as many of the interview panel as is possible at least with eye contact and perhaps a small nod. If the panel is very large this will not be possible. Do not look at the floor or stare blankly at the wall behind the chairman of the panel. Do not sit down until you are invited to do so.

If somebody—probably the chairman—shakes your hand, then try to meet his handshake with one of equal force. Don't counter his firm grasp with a limp-wristed effort, and if he is a rather frail individual with a gentle touch, do not assume that crushing his metacarpo-phalangeal joints with a vigorous response will win you any friends. If you happen to be a member of any curious societies who use a characteristic 'secret' handshake, then do *not* use it in the interview. Either it will go unnoticed and so will be of no benefit, or, in the unlikely event that the recipient of your handshake is a member of the same mysterious society, it might be perceived as a feeble effort to gain an unfair advantage in the proceedings, and this will act against you.

When you do sit, try to avoid giving the impression of a captured soldier undergoing interrogation. It is reasonable to turn the chair to a slight angle and to sit with your legs crossed if you wish, with your hands on your lap. Try to avoid looking terrified or gripping the arms of the chair tightly. Do not, under any circumstances, adopt a posture that could be regarded as 'slouching'. If the chair is a relatively comfy chair with a low back, sometimes this can be difficult, and you may wish to sit forward on the edge of the chair. The overriding goal is to give an air of cool professionalism.

EYE CONTACT, WHERE TO LOOK AND THE 'CV RUN-THROUGH'

Virtually all medical job interviews begin the same way, and that is the chairman of the panel will introduce you to all the other members of the panel. Frequently, you will know these individuals since you may have been working with them already, or you may have recently had lengthy discussions with them regarding the reasons why you want this job. No matter how well you know the panel you must 'play a straight bat' from this point onwards. It may be the case that somebody interviewing you is one of your regular drinking or mountaineering partners but that fact will not be known to other members of the panel, and excessive informality simply goes down very badly. An interview is a formal occasion and you must behave appropriately. Therefore, when each member of the panel is introduced it is reasonable to nod and say, 'hello', but probably no more than that. Once the introductions are completed the chairman of the interview panel will almost certainly hand straight over to the representative of the Royal College or, alternatively, another member of the panel who will start going through your CV.

Bear in mind at this point that although every word of your CV is known to you and undoubtedly you will be able to recite it verbatim, it is possible that the panel member now holding your CV may never have seen it before. So, although you may think it is obvious that your career progression during the past 6 years is written down with impeccable clarity, the person now looking at your hieroglyphics may not find it quite so clear. You need to nod and make small comments of agreement as this panel member starts going through your CV noting where you went to school, where you trained, where you did your house jobs, where you did your SHO or FY2 rotation and so on.

While this panel member is doing this task he is totting up in his head the number of months you have spent in each job, basically satisfying himself that you have done the right amount of previous training to be suitable for the present post. Frequently, this adding up procedure goes wrong and it is perfectly reasonable for you to politely interrupt and correct the panel member if his sums are going awry. Be ready at this point to have answers to questions regarding what you did during any obvious gaps in your professional training. You may think that your CV clearly indicates the 4 months that you spent at a mission hospital in central Africa, but it may not be immediately evident to the Royal College representative struggling to find his way around your CV, and you need to be ready to help if necessary. Try to avoid getting into lengthy discussions regarding what you have or have not done in the past at this point, since this early part of the interview is very much an assessment to check that you are suitable for the job in question. Also, be absolutely certain that you can recall every detail of your own training progression since candidates who struggle to remember exactly where they did their first SHO or FY2 job can look very silly indeed in front of interview panels.

Once this initial 'CV run-through' has been completed, the chairman of the interview panel will invite other members of the panel to question you in turn. It is possible that not all the members of the interview panel will ask questions. The actual questions that you may be asked are dealt with in other sections of this book, but in starting to consider how to deal with the questions two general principles apply. The first of these is that whatever question you are asked you must try to give your answers promptly, brightly and using the guiding principle of 'cool professionalism with sparkle'. Your style of answering should be confident, polite, to the point and yet not bland. A brief reflective moment to gather your thoughts before you start to speak is fine, but avoid absolutely any prolonged 'pregnant pauses'. Remember that although this interview is the most important thing that has happened to you for many months, for the members of the panel it may be something of a chore and you may be the eighth candidate that they have interviewed that afternoon. Therefore, a degree of enthusiasm and sparkle must come through in all your answers to draw the attention of the panel to you and to gain their interest.

The second guiding principle for answering interview questions is related, and is this: although just one member of the panel will have asked you the question, you need to deliver your answer to *all* the members of the panel. In other words, although you should start by facing the questioner and beginning your answer, as you develop your reply you should engage in eye contact with other members of the panel, turning your head if necessary, to make sure that the right side of the room is not bored if the question came from the left side of the panel and vice versa. Your goal is to impress not just the person who has asked you the question but to make sure that you win over every member of the panel with every answer to every question. The art of head turning and gaining eye contact with others is not one which doctors practice. Watch politicians delivering a speech to a large audience. They do it well. That is because they have been trained, and it is quite reasonable for you to train yourself by asking some friends to give you a mock interview. If there are two or three of them make them sit in different areas of the room and practice getting all of them involved with your answers to their questions.

GESTURE

Many interview candidates sit with their hands firmly clasped together or, worse still, their arms folded throughout the whole interview. This is a disaster and gives a very bad impression to the panel. Again, observe a politician being interviewed on television; watch how they use their hands. Seldom is there any wild, expansive gesture but very frequently there is small reinforcement of points that they are making by using small gestures with one hand. This is something that you should practice. Also, panels are very impressed with a reasoned answer containing several components, each thread of which is enumerated by tapping one finger on to the fingers of the opposite hand as though you were counting. Simple gesture makes for a good delivery and can be surprisingly effective at making one candidate 'stand out from the crowd'. Gesture should be subtle and restrained but should be used. Just be careful not to overdo it and ensure that you don't turn the whole thing into a sort of game of charades.

VOICE USAGE

A medical job interview is not the correct forum in which to rehearse your imitation of Richard Burton or Laurence Olivier, at least not unless your natural voice already sounds like one of them. All the same, it is worth considering before the event how you use your voice in an interview, in order to avoid disasters. For example, make sure that you do not deliver your answers like some interviewees who have an alarming tendency to drop the volume of their voice lower and lower as they speak, so that the members of the interview panel are required to lean further and further forward in their seats in order to hear what is being said.

If you have absorbed the messages given elsewhere in this book, you will know that there is a very real benefit to be gained by saying answers to 'predictable questions' out loud before the interview. Ask one of your friends to listen to you when you do so, and ask them how you sound. Most theatre and film actors will experiment many times with the manner in which they deliver a given line, and there is no reason why you should not experiment by rehearsing answers to questions in different styles beforehand. Work out which type of voice usage you feel most comfortable using.

If you feel that everything you say sounds terrible, then try sitting up straighter, opening your mouth wider, and aim to get more energy into your voice. Imagine that you have just been to the cinema and seen the best film you've seen for many years and you're describing it enthusiastically to a close friend. Think about the way you would use your voice doing that, and then use the same voice to practise delivering answers to potential interview questions. You will almost certainly sound significantly better. Remember that your goal is not just to be heard, your goal is to make an impact!

Have you ever wondered whether your *speed* of talking is correct? If so, then the answer is that it will almost certainly be too fast. If you are in any doubt at all, then *slow it down*! It is very unlikely that you will speak too slowly in the interview, but many candidates—particularly women—speak far too quickly.

HOW TO END THE INTERVIEW

When the interview is over and all the questions have been asked then you will be invited to leave. This instruction may be preceded by the chairman of the panel letting you know that they will come to a decision perhaps later that day, in which case he may invite you to wait. Alternatively, he may suggest that the decision will not be made until the following day, in which case he will ask whether the secretary of the panel has appropriate contact details for you. Make up your mind in advance whether you are going to stay to hear the result if it is only going to be an hour or so later. In general terms interview panels like to be able to greet the successful candidate at the end of the afternoon, so stay if you can. However, if you have travelled a long distance and have a train or plane to catch to return home, then they will not be irritated if you ask them to contact you by telephone with news of the outcome.

When you stand from your chair do not blindly walk out of the room but make a point of acknowledging as many members of the panel as possible with a small nod and the single phrase, 'thank you', addressed to the panel as a whole. Then leave, trying to ensure that you know which way the door of the interview room opens to avoid unnecessary pulling when you should be pushing. You must also make absolutely certain that you do not use the wrong door and unintentionally exit into the broom cupboard, thus generating an embarrassing scene with any pretence of 'cool professionalism' being irretrievably lost.

POINTS FOR REFLECTION

- Have you practised delivering interview answers?
- Are you able to organise a mock interview?
- If you've already done a mock interview, how did it go? Do you need to try it again?

SPECIFIC INTERVIEW STRATEGIES

chapter 9

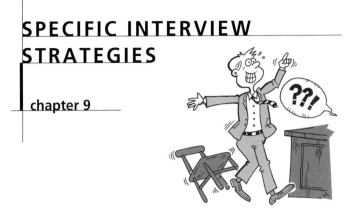

At the start of this book, we suggested that getting yourself onto the shortlist should be viewed as something akin to a military operation. Once you are in the interview itself, however, there is generally no need for such covert manoeuvering, and you can simply be yourself, answering questions with professionalism and enthusiasm. Sometimes, though, you may have a suspicion before the interview that you are in a certain position 'in the running', and under these circumstances it is occasionally worth modifying your approach very slightly.

'I'M IN THERE ALREADY'

If you really know before the event that you are the 'front runner' (and, of course, this would be a very happy position in which to be), then your biggest risk is that you somehow 'blow it'. Therefore, make sure that you handle the interview in a smooth, professional, and orthodox way. By all means

Getting that Medical Job: Secrets for Success, 3rd edition. © Colin J. Mumford and Suvankar Pal. Published 2011 by Blackwell Publishing Ltd.

be animated and enthusiastic, but make sure that you don't 'overtalk' or start to deliver an unnecessary lecture mid-interview which may run the risk of alienating one or more members of the panel.

Give well-considered and thoughtful answers to questions, avoiding controversy, and keep in the back of your mind that all you have to do is *confirm* to the panel that you are the right person for the job. Do not risk losing the backing of people who may already be your main supporters by saying anything in-flammatory or very unexpected, and above all do not be flip-pant. In other words, play the interview with a 'straight bat'.

THE RANK OUTSIDER

The situation is different if you know that you are an outsider and way down the list of likely winners. Under these circum-stances a 'straight bat' interview is fine, but is very unlikely to get you the job. Therefore, you may want to risk a much more aggressive stance, and deliver a so-called 'machine gun inter-view'. This style of interview technique aims to leave a panel saying 'Wow!' when you leave the room, and gets your name mentioned in the consideration of the 'final few' when the panel start their deliberations.

The trick is for you to be noticeably more dynamic than all the other candidates, with imaginative and possibly even rather 'whacky' answers to questions. Some answers you give might be deliberately provocative to try to get the panel engaged in a robust discussion with you. It is also fine in this style of in-terviewing to offer answers to questions which many people would consider out-of-line with majority opinion on a subject, provided you can justify and expand on what you are saying. Smile a lot, really trying to engage every panel member, and try to come over as an individual with a great passion and strength of feelings about the subjects raised. The hope is that one or two members of the panel may be attracted to someone whom they feel is 'more sparky' than the rest of the field, and they might just offer you the job. Bear in mind, however, that this is a very 'high-risk' strategy, and it may well fail. So only consider this sort of approach if you know that the interview is unlikely to lead to success!

UNORTHODOXY

With the exception of the 'machine gun interview' strategy described above, be very careful about unorthodoxy in an interview; in other words, don't be too unconventional or say things that are a long way out of line with accepted opinion. This rule extends to what you wear and how you enter and leave the room, as well as to what you say in response to questions. Some degree of 'distinguishing style' in an interview is fine, and the odd controversial answer to a question is usually okay, provided you make some acknowledgement that you realise your own view is not matched by others, and you can defend yourself if the panel picks up on what you have said. Often the attention of a panel is aroused by presentation of non-standard views and unexpected answers to questions, particularly if they are interviewing a large series of candidates. But remember that you are not there to provide an entertaining interlude for those people interviewing, you are there to get the job!

LYING

This issue requires a very simple instruction: 'don't do it!' You may think that you can gloss over the 6-month 'unfilled gap' on your curriculum vitae that arose because you were on a course and badly failed the exam at the end of it; but if the panel question you about that period of time, then you should simply tell them what happened. Many people have mishaps and exam failures during the course of a medical career, and by and large interview panels are not too troubled by them. However, they *will* be troubled—intensely—if they perceive that a candidate in an interview is lying to them, and it will undoubtedly guarantee failure. Even worse, if it were the case that a candidate claims to have a postgraduate qualification that they do not possess, then this becomes yet more serious, and is likely to threaten any further progression of that doctor's career, with involvement of the General Medical Council, other regulatory authorities and formal disciplinary procedures. *Do not lie in interviews!*

POINT FOR REFLECTION

• What strategy will you be adopting in your own interview?

THE QUESTIONS: GENERAL POINTS

chapter 10

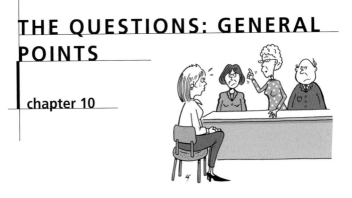

One very important mistake that interview candidates make is they fail to realise that it is entirely feasible to work out what questions you will be asked in the interview long before you ever find yourself sitting in front of the panel. Many candidates do not believe that such a feat is possible. However, the sequence of questions which is asked in a medical job interview, regardless of the grade of post being applied for, and particularly when interviewing candidates for specialty training posts, is remarkably consistent. Some of these have already been considered in previous sections of this book. Even at senior levels, to a great extent the flow of questions that a candidate will be asked when applying for a consultant-grade job can also be largely anticipated in advance. In other words, some questions are inevitable.

INEVITABLE QUESTIONS

With some thought it is very easy to see what the 'inevitable' questions will be. If, for example, you are applying to be a

Getting that Medical Job: Secrets for Success, 3rd edition. © Colin J. Mumford and Suvankar Pal. Published 2011 by Blackwell Publishing Ltd.

specialty trainee in gastroenterology in a major city in the Midlands then you will undoubtedly be asked, first, 'why gastroenterology?' and, secondly, 'why this city?' Whether you like the thought of these questions or not you are under an absolute obligation to have clear, well thought out and concise answers to both of these. Remember, when you frame your answers that all the time the essence is not just to show that you are good at answering these questions. The overwhelming priority is to show through your answers that you are unequivocally the best person for the job. Any sort of rambling or waffling answer to these first questions, for example comments such as 'Well, I'm really not sure what I want to do, but I think gastroenterology seems like a good idea' is a recipe for disaster. Equally, when considering the city in which you have applied to work, remember that the unit in that city may have been the product of years and years of work by the members of the panel who are now interviewing you, and comments such as, 'Well, I thought I'd try here first because the advert was the first to appear in the *British Medical Journal*, but I'm equally enthusiastic about cities X and Y' is not the sort of answer that builds up warmth between the interview panel and you.

You need to frame and construct your answers with some care, and it would be our suggestion that you adhere to the guiding principle suggested in previous sections of this book, which could loosely be described as 'cool professionalism with enthusiasm'. You must show that, first, you are perfectly capable as a doctor, secondly, that you will be capable of performing brilliantly in the post which is on offer and, thirdly, demonstrate that you are entirely professional about all you do. However, your answers must have a certain gloss—a kind of sparkle—which demonstrates an enthusiasm which is often not shown by the candidates against whom you will be competing. Therefore, let 'cool professionalism with enthusiasm' be in the back of your mind whilst you are delivering your answers.

Remember that the interview panel will like to feel that some praise is being offered for their unit through the medium of your answers. Therefore, a good answer dealing with the question 'Why do you want to come to this city?' might include observations such as: 'You have to look a long way to find a training programme in gastroenterology which is as well constructed and offers such good variety as the post in this city. There are very few other centres that allow a rotation between hospitals giving me a chance to work with a number of different consultants in the field, all of whom have differing subspecialty interests.'

You can then add other riders to your comments according to the specific circumstances of the post for which you have applied; for example, 'Of particular appeal in the present post is the close liaison which you enjoy with, (e.g.) the regional liver transplant programme, since this is an area of gastroenterology that particularly interests me.' Or you might add, for example, 'The present post is particularly exciting because of the high intensity emergency work which is done and the close links which you have with the supra-regional trauma centre which is on this site.' All the time your answers must be focused and enthusiastic making it quite plain that no other job is the one for you except for the present job which is on offer.

It is only in interviews at a relatively junior level that you can expect to be asked 'Why this subject?' and, again, your answers must be well thought out and show total enthusiasm and commitment to the specialty which you are trying to enter.

A word of caution is necessary at this point for the candidate who is applying for a specialist registrar or a consultant job in a location *in which he is already working*. In a previous section of this book, we have drawn attention to the grave risk that candidates who are well known to the panel may be excessively informal and sometimes even flippant with an interview panel made up of senior doctors whom they already know well. This is a great mistake and is to be avoided at all costs. This scenario also gives rise to a question which may floor an unwary candidate and that is something along the lines of: 'Surely, having worked with us for the past 12 months you cannot possibly want to carry on working with us for the next 5 or 6 years?' This sometimes comes as an unexpected question for a candidate and a clear answer, again avoiding inappropriate humour or flippancy, is necessary. Our suggestion would be to turn the question on its head and use it to your advantage by saying something along the lines of: 'It is precisely because I have had the opportunity of working in this department and with several members of the panel that I realise exactly what an excellent opportunity for further training in gastroenterology this unit offers. I have had the opportunity to take part in the inpatient and outpatient service as well as helping to shape our present emergency service, and I very much want to develop these aspects of the service in the next stage of my career.'

It would be perfectly reasonable to add (whether you believe it or not): 'Indeed, having had the opportunity to compare my experience in this department with colleagues who have worked in other departments, I can see that there are few other departments around the country that can offer (e. g.) a specialist registrar position with so many exciting opportunities as the present post.' And you could conclude this rather difficult moment in the interview by reinforcing the point, '. . .so it is *because* I am already familiar with the department that I am so excited and enthusiastic about the post which is on offer.'

PROBABLE QUESTIONS

Some of the questions that are listed above can be guaranteed to be asked in just about every medical interview. There will then follow a series of questions which can also largely be anticipated. If you are applying for a post at a relatively junior level you will be asked about your experience of the clinical training course in your medical school, how much time you spent in general medicine, general surgery, accident and emergency and so on. Most interview panellists who will be genuinely interested in the medical curricula at other medical schools may well ask a question along the lines of: 'If you were planning your own medical curriculum what would you alter?' There is no right or wrong answer to this, but a thoughtful answer which makes sense to the interview panellist will usually go down well.

In framing an answer to this sort of a question you should be prepared to provoke a little discussion with the panel and don't worry if they seem to disagree with some of your observations; stick to your guns and say why you would change the curriculum in the way that you have proposed. The only wrong way to answer the question is to spend a long time 'umming' and 'aaahing' and then say something rather limp like, 'Well I thought our course was probably alright, I don't think anything needs changing.' This sort of answer loses the feeling of enthusiasm which you are trying to convey.

Again, if you are applying for a post at a junior level you can be certain that some time will be spent asking about your elective period. Be sure that you know exactly where you went, and if you worked with anybody famous, who they were, since it is possible that they will be known to the panel. Conversely, if you went somewhere exotic, for example, the Caribbean and spent the whole 8-week period playing golf, lying on the beach and windsurfing, then do *not* say this in your answer. Whilst many interview panels will realise that this is a very important part of student elective periods, they will not wish to be told so in the formal environment of an interview, and you must therefore be prepared to talk about the difficulties of delivering community paediatric care in remote areas of Caribbean islands or something similar. Remember that you are showing 'cool professionalism' all the time. Whilst one or two members of the panel may, themselves, be enthusiastic golfers or windsurfers, they will not wish to hear that this was the way in which you spent your elective period.

Research and publications are a guaranteed part of any interview. If you have had the skill to produce an undergraduate publication and you are applying for a junior-level post, then undergraduate publications greatly impress the panel, and you may be surprised to be asked about this in some detail. Therefore, you must be able to quote the title of any papers which resulted from your work and you should have prepared a short paragraph in your head, which will explain in simple terms to individuals who are not familiar with your field, what you did and why your research was of interest. Remember at this point the lay member on the panel; in other words, remember that your answer must be intelligible to somebody who may not know any medicine at all. Sometimes, interview candidates at both junior and senior level are quite incapable of explaining the nature of their research work in a simple way to people who are very experienced in medicine but not familiar with the specific area of research. If you cannot explain your own research in a simple way to an interview panel, then they will lose interest in your answer and, at the same time that they lose interest in your answer, they will also lose interest in you.

It is worth stressing a second 'guiding principle' at this point and that is many interview candidates believe that it is up to them to show that 'they are right for the job'. Curiously, this is not necessarily the overriding goal in an interview because it could be argued that everybody who has found their way onto the shortlist is 'right for the job'. If they were not 'right for the job' then they would not have been shortlisted in the first place. So, a second thought needs to be in the back of your mind as you are delivering all your answers during the interview, namely you need to show the panel that 'not only are you right for the job, *but the job is right for you at this stage in your career*'. This assertion requires a little thought, but it is very true that there is often little to choose between interview candidates who have been shortlisted for a given post, and in the discussion which follows 'behind closed doors' after all candidates have been interviewed, a decision which may seem to be very diffi-cult indeed can sometimes be resolved by the interview panel deciding the answer to the question: 'For which of the candi-dates whom we have just interviewed is this job the most ap-propriate at this stage in their career?' Therefore, if you—when delivering your answers—have stressed the point that not only are you the right, most appropriate person for the job, but also that the job is clearly the right way that you 'should be moving' at this stage in your career progression, then that message may hit home, and getting that point across is frequently the single best way to win over an interview panel. Panels do not like indi-viduals that seem to be 'drifting' from one job to the next. They are far more impressed by an individual who has 'nailed their colours to the mast' and who has demonstrated a clear career di-rection. Part of that demonstration means that you need to show the panel that the job is right for you at this moment in time.

PROBLEM QUESTIONS AND HOW TO ESCAPE

There are a number of 'sticky moments' which often crop up in interviews and rather surprisingly some of these can also be an-ticipated and a way out identified. It is often sensible to have identified the escape routes from these 'sticky' interview mo-ments before you are faced with them in front of a formal panel. The following are some examples.

You've done no research

Most hospital specialists need to do research. Certainly, they need to have published a few papers before getting to senior level. Some individuals are wonderful clinicians and seem to get a long way up the career ladder without doing any research at all. The time this matters is when they are faced with an in-terview panel. If your CV is short on publications and original research, then you need to have some sort of an answer ready in case this issue is brought up. Rather than meekly admitting that you are a failure when it comes to writing papers, it is better to try and turn this shortcoming into a strength, perhaps by saying something like: 'You will see from my CV that my greatest strengths are in the field of clinical medicine. My whole career so far has been very much orientated towards a clinical progression rather than a research or academic approach. I think my greatest contribution has been in liaison with my research colleagues and providing a source of patients and clinical ideas to enhance their own research. Therefore, I feel I have contributed to a number of different research projects over the years, but *as a clinician*, and I have not been the major author of any of the resulting publications.' This may or may not be true but an answer along these lines is at least an attempt to turn a weakness into a strength.

You're applying for a 5-year rotation but the whole panel knows that you really want to go and work in Australia as soon as possible

Many junior doctors express enthusiasm to spend 1 or 2 years abroad at some point during their career and there is no need to hide this fact during the interview. The concern that worries interview panels most is if they think a new appointee is going to leave within a few months of arriving in a post since then a replacement will need to be found very quickly, and that does not go down well. You do not, however, need to keep the fact that you are thinking of doing a year or two abroad a secret, but it is reasonable to give your overseas intentions a rather low profile, and to take an approach along the lines of: 'Although I have said for some time I would be interested in exploring the possibility of working overseas for a year or two, my major interest is to get an excellent training (e. g.) in gastroenterology, and the present post offers me the chance of getting such a training. Therefore, my prime enthusiasm is to gain appointment to the present job and work my way through this rotation for a number of years. It may be in years to come I will think about exploring the possibility of a year abroad, but that would only be with the full agreement of the senior colleagues with whom I was working at that time.'

You don't really want the job but your boyfriend/girlfriend/wife/husband works in this city

Candidates are often surprised that interview panels are remarkably human. Therefore, if you have pressing social, domestic or family reasons why you want to work in this city, then it is quite acceptable to say so. If you are a total 'no-hoper', then a plea that your boyfriend or girlfriend lives and works in this city is unlikely to secure you the job. However, if you are running neck and neck with one of the other candidates and you have a crucial domestic reason why you would like to come to this particular city, then that is often influential when it comes to decision time. Accordingly, you do not need to be afraid of mentioning your social situation as one reason for wanting to work in a specific location. Comments in that regard, however, *must* be linked with the sorts of answers offered in paragraphs above, indicating a strong enthusiasm for the post, the training that is offered, the individuals with whom you would be working and so on.

It's far too early in your career for the job that you are applying for but you are 'chancing your arm'

This is a difficult issue and interview panels will often identify this problem very quickly. Occasionally, extreme enthusiasm and confidence both before and during the interview will win the day here. This problem is actually less frequent following the introduction of a more regimented training system for specialist registrars in the United Kingdom, since this system now dictates that candidates must have done a certain amount of general professional training at foundation year level before they are allowed to enter the specialty training grades, and at the end of the specialist registrar period there is now a strictly-defined time period during which specialist registrars may start to look for their consultant job.

Nevertheless, it sometimes happens that a relatively junior foundation year doctor wants to apply for the perfect specialist registrar rotation in the very best centre, and, in our view, it is quite reasonable to make every effort to get that job since the chance may not come around again for very many years. You must then be prepared to take a relatively aggressive stance in an interview making it quite plain that you feel very confident in your ability to perform well in the job for which you are applying. You need to show that you have masses of experience in the short time that you have been in the foundation training years and that you have made a great effort to get to know the new hospital, unit and ward in which you will be working. You need to stress repeatedly during your answers that you feel 'entirely confident that you would be able to perform the job appropriately', but bear in mind your answers must not be so aggressive as to sound 'cocky' or overconfident. If you really feel that the post on offer is the chance of a lifetime then by all means say so in the interview, since this will continue the air of *professionalism with enthusiasm*, which is so important in ensuring success.

You're really not sure if you want this job or not

This is an issue that we addressed in the first section of this book. There is simply no excuse for sitting in an interview for a job which you are not totally certain that you want. Of course, you *may* apply for a job and then withdraw prior to the interview. Even if you find yourself in the horrible situation that you are in front of the interview panel and then decide that you really do not want the job, then you should say so and explain your reasons why. The real catastrophe is when individuals do well in an interview, are offered the job, and then decline the job a couple of days—or worse still—a couple of weeks later. This generates intense animosity on the part of interview panels who will then have to be reconvened in order to appoint another candidate. It will potentially wreck your career because word gets around that you have 'dropped out after appointment' and there is certainly a chance that your referees will be contacted and an explanation will be demanded as to why you have behaved in the way that you have. Therefore, if you are not 100% certain that you want this job, make sure that you are not in the interview in the first place!

'CRINGE' QUESTIONS

Medical interviews are different from many other sorts of interview. Some people see them as more challenging than the interviews which our colleagues in industry face; others see them as very much lighter than the gruelling interviews faced by professionals in other walks of life. For example, if you were being interviewed for a post outside the world of medicine you might find yourself being asked a series of rather curious questions, for example: 'What are your strengths?', 'What are your weaknesses?', 'What is your greatest achievement?'. These are questions which most medical students and doctors would not find easy to answer at the best of times, yet they sometimes, albeit infrequently, crop up in medical interviews. They usually come from a panel member who cannot think of anything better to ask, and occasionally they come from the lay member of the panel. These are sometimes rather irreverently referred to as 'cringe questions'. They're given that name because not only will you cringe when the question is posed, but virtually every other member of the interview panel will also inwardly cringe with embarrassment. So you need to get through these questions as quickly as possible, whilst at the same time not saying anything incriminating. Most of us could offer a fair answer to the question 'What are your strengths?' and an answer such as: 'I'm a hard worker, I'm enthusiastic in what I do, and most people say that I am very easy to get on with' is perfectly adequate, and is quite long enough.

Rather harder is framing an answer to the question: 'What are your weaknesses?' On occasion one of the authors has heard candidates offer astonishingly foolish answers to this question which immediately excluded them from any chance of success in the interview. For example, statements such as: 'Well, sometimes I find it impossible to get out of bed in the morning', or worse still: 'Well, I think I have a tendency to upset the nursing staff on my ward', reveal commendable frankness but are catastrophic in terms of securing success in the interview. We suggest that the only suitable answer for the 'weakness' question needs to be something that allows the rest of the panel to chuckle and get over their embarrassment quickly. A good answer might be: 'Well, I have to confess that I am obsessively punctual and completely intolerant of slothfulness', ideally delivered with a wry smile around the table. This sort of thing allows everybody on the panel to relax again.

As regards your 'greatest achievement', then few of us would feel that anything that we have done in medicine really rates as 'our greatest achievement'. If, however, you single-handedly ran a paediatric surgical unit in the middle of rural Africa during your student elective period, then it might be reasonable to say so at this point. If you do not have an obvious medical achievement which is breathtaking, it is often better to retreat to a rather endearing answer and reply with something like: 'Being awarded my 50 metres swimming certificate at the age of 5' or 'Receiving an invitation to give a solo organ recital in the local cathedral, following a successful school concert.'

'GOOGLIES'

Sometimes an interview panel member will throw a very un-expected and rather difficult question at you. It may be a con-fusing question or may seem to be needlessly aggressive. They are doing this for a reason, and that is simply to see whether you are able to spark and cope when put under a bit of pres-sure. These questions are sometimes referred to as 'googlies'. It does not happen very often but you need to be prepared for the sort of question that goes: 'I see that you have just spent 6 months working in Sunnydale Accident and Emergency unit. Everybody knows that that unit is totally useless and should be closed down forthwith. Don't you agree?' Remember that the other interview panellists will be surprised at hearing a ques-tion like this from one of their colleagues, and therefore this can work to your favour. The interest of the interview panel will suddenly have been aroused and you can maintain their interest by being equally robust in your answer which might be along the lines of: 'No, I totally disagree. I am aware of the rumours circulating regarding the Sunnydale casualty service but hav-ing worked there very recently I find these stories astonishing. They are totally unfounded. Furthermore, I would suggest that some of the work practices which we employ at Sunnydale are streets ahead of the services offered at comparable units. I think that the people making these criticisms should come and spend some time with us and see exactly what they could learn from the set-up at Sunnydale.'

You may get other questions that are less aggressive but equally likely to fox the unwary candidate. For example: 'If the centre of Birmingham were hit by a nuclear bomb tomorrow and all the hospitals at which you have been working during the past 5 years were destroyed, how would you rebuild them? Would it be one huge hospital or several small ones?' Obviously, there is no right or wrong answer to this sort of question but panels will be genuinely interested in your view. Any sort of well thought out plan to redevelop health services in Birmingham would be an acceptable answer. A bad answer would be something along the lines of: 'Well, I don't really know—I've never really put much thought into how hospitals function. I wouldn't be able to plan for a project like that.' This sort of feeble answer lacks enthusiasm and lacks sparkle.

HANDLING THE LAY MEMBER OF THE PANEL

You may well be asked questions by the lay panel member. It is an unfortunate fact that most of the other members of the interview panel will be rather less interested in the questions that come to you from this individual, and probably less interested in your answers. Therefore, your answers need to be polite, enthusiastic but very much to the point. For example, if it says on your CV that you write children's books in Welsh then it is almost a running certainty that the lay member of the panel will want to spend some time talking to you about this. You need to be focused and crisp in your answers. This is because although it may be of great personal interest to you that you have achieved such literary success in Wales, it will not, however, be of any great interest to the rest of the interview panel. Your answers will give little clue as to whether you are or are not capable of doing the medical job for which you have applied. So you need to smile, be polite, but keep your answers relatively short when it comes to the lay member of the panel. Remember all the time that you are trying to show cool professionalism with enthusiasm and that 'cool professionalism' means professionalism as a medic not as a children's author. In your answers aim to keep coming back to your great enthusiasm for the medical subject for which you are applying. Avoid at all costs starting giving a mini-lecture on a non-medical subject to which you devote your spare time.

HILL WALKING AND MOTORBIKES

On your CV there will be a section headed 'interests', and towards the end of the interview one or other member of the panel will ask you something about your hobbies. The guiding principle here is similar to the principle which must be adopted when handling the lay panel member in that you need to be aware that there is a risk of becoming involved in a rather lengthy, and inappropriate, discussion on diverse aspects of hill climbing, mountaineering equipment and so on. This may be of interest to the odd member of the panel who knows something about the sport, but will be of virtually no interest to any other member of the panel, all of whom will be getting bored at this stage in the interview. Therefore, if you are an enthusiastic hill walker or motorcyclist it is perfectly reasonable to say so, perhaps commenting in a sentence or two on the problems faced by the British motorcycle industry in the face of competition from the Japanese. However, do not get bogged down in this, since that it is not what you are in a medical interview for. You can save that sort of discussion for the celebratory beer once you are successful after the interview.

'ANY QUESTIONS FOR THE PANEL...?'

In the same way that you can predict the opening questions in a medical interview, you can guarantee what the final question will be. The chairman of the panel will look at his colleagues and then will turn to you and will say something along the lines of: 'Well, that is all the questions we have for you. I wonder if you have any questions for us?' What, in fact, the chairman of the panel is saying is that in their opinion the panel feel that the interview is now at an end. They wish to see the back of you and start on the next candidate. All of them are probably hoping that you will *not* have 'any questions for the panel'. Moreover, if you do have questions that you want to put to the panel now is not the right time to do it. You should have done it before the interview, and if you have overlooked anything then you should sort it out afterwards.

We suggest, therefore, that there is only one suitable answer to this question and that is something along the lines of: 'Thank you, but no. I have had the chance of meeting several members of the panel in advance of this interview and all my questions have been answered. Thank you.' And at that point you shut up. Somebody will then stand up and show you the way to the door. That is the time to leave.

THE QUESTIONS: ACTUAL QUESTIONS AND ANSWERS

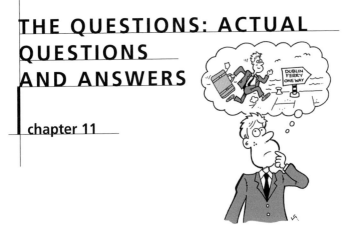

chapter 11

GOOD, BAD AND GHASTLY

The last chapter of this book considered some general issues surrounding the range and breadth of questions asked in a medical job interview. It is now worth looking at some specific examples. In an ideal world, a book like this would include a computerised CD-ROM which would contain recordings of actual questions asked and the answers given, in a genuine interview situation. Unfortunately, rules regarding the confidentiality of what is said during an interview prevent such an inclusion. But some actual questions and answers have been presented in earlier chapters of this book, and in the paragraphs which follow we give a few more examples of real questions asked, and the answers given by candidates, heard by the authors and some of our colleagues during medical job interviews. These are not, strictly speaking, word-for-word reproductions of what was said, and in most instances we have

Getting that Medical Job: Secrets for Success, 3rd edition. © Colin J. Mumford and Suvankar Pal. Published 2011 by Blackwell Publishing Ltd.

slightly changed the form of words used in order to preserve confidentiality, but these examples are illustrative.

It will be appreciated that many of these questions fall into the categories of 'cringe questions' and 'googlies' referred to previously. We've made some comments after each one.

Questioner (in a consultant interview): 'Looking at your CV, I would say that you'd be far more suited to a career in research and academia. Why you are applying for a full-time NHS post?'

Candidate (unsuccessful): 'Research is too much like hard work in my view.'

This answer fell into the category of excessive and inappropriate honesty together with a degree of flippancy. A priority in any medical interview is the recognition that it is a formal situation, and particularly in a consultant-level interview, jocularity in dealing with a question like this was not appropriate. With a little thought, the candidate could have framed a far more impressive and reasonable answer.

Questioner (specialist registrar interview): 'I'd like you to choose one adjective that describes yourself. What is it?'

Candidate (successful): 'Approachable.'

This was undoubtedly a 'cringe question', and most members of the panel took a small intake of breath when it was asked. Nevertheless, it seems to be a question which is relatively frequently used both in medical interviews and elsewhere. The answer that the successful candidate gave was a good one, because it was novel and thoughtful, and it followed a series of weaker answers from other candidates, including predictable ones such as 'enthusiastic', 'keen' and 'friendly', and the dreadful answer, 'Gosh, that's difficult, I can't think of anything.'

Questioner (specialist registrar interview): 'I'd like you to pick one paper which you have recently read in a medical journal. Tell me about it.'

Candidate (unsuccessful): 'I can't think of one.'

This question fell into the category of 'predictable questions', and the answer was unforgivable. Every candidate for a hospital doctor post should at least have some idea of what has appeared in the medical journals in the weeks prior to their interview. Even if the candidate had not been able to comment on a specific scientific paper, he could at least have discussed an interesting editorial in one of the medical journals or, if all else failed, steered the question to talking about a medical piece in the national press.

Questioner (in an specialist registrar interview, to an Irish doctor): 'I see that you're Irish, and you trained in Ireland. Isn't it a well-known fact that all Irish graduates inevitably return to Ireland in the long run, so why should we give you postgraduate training here?'

Candidate (successful): 'That's not true at all! Whilst it may be the case that many Irish doctors who have been junior hospital doctors in Ireland come to Britain for a while and then go back straight after their registrar post, you'll see from my CV that I left Ireland at the end of my first postgraduate year and have worked in the United Kingdom ever since then. I have every intention of remaining in Britain for the foreseeable future and when I eventually apply for my consultant post I'll make a decision at that stage whether I want to stay in Britain or go back to Ireland.'

This question could be classed as a 'googly'. The questioner was presumably being deliberately provocative to see how the candidate reacted. It was a robust, fair and sensible answer.

Questioner (in a research registrar interview): 'Do you think that all hospital doctors should spend a period of time in research?'

Candidate (successful): 'No. I have a large number of colleagues who aim to become hospital consultants. Some of them are obviously well-suited to research whereas others are not. Some of these others would be far better placed, and of more use to their eventual employer, if they spent a period of time gaining, for example, an MBA degree. I think there probably should be more alternatives in the medical career ladder to the traditional 2- or 3-year period of research.'

There was no right or wrong answer to this question. The candidate said what he thought and presented his views well.

Questioner (in a specialist registrar interview where two posts at two different centres were on offer): 'You know that there are two posts on offer at the moment. I see that you have only applied for one of them. What's wrong with the post at my hospital?'

Candidate (successful): 'Of course there is nothing wrong with the post at your hospital, and all things being equal I would have applied for both posts. Unfortunately, if I were appointed to the post in your centre, I would be geographically disadvantaged, because my boyfriend lives in the other city.'

The questioner presented this question in a slightly cheeky way. The candidate responded in similar vein and generated some humour among the interview panel when she used the phrase 'geographically disadvantaged'. It was a perfectly reasonable explanation for why she had applied for only one of the two posts on offer.

Questioner (specialist registrar interview): 'There are six candidates for this job sitting outside the door, all of whom have similar CVs. Why should we have you?'

Candidate (unsuccessful): 'Well, err...I suppose I get on okay with people, I'm reliable and will do the work. Otherwise I don't really know.'

The answer to this question began fairly badly and then got even worse. A question like this demands a punchy, well-prepared and unequivocal answer that leaves the panel no option other than to appoint. In this example, the candidate began in a slightly self-effacing manner, and then ended extremely limply. All candidates should have a powerful ready response to this question to show the panel why they are 'the best'.

Questioner (old-style senior house officer interview): 'I see that you've just taken 12 months off for a round-the-world yacht race. Surely that was a complete waste of time?'

Candidate (successful): 'In the past 12 months I've learnt a fantastic range of skills. Specifically, I've learnt how to work in a team and I've learnt a great deal about man management. I've also had to keep my head in extremely testing and demanding situations where there was potential for catastrophe if things went wrong. I'm certain that skills like these can only help the progress of my medical career.'

Once again, this was a slightly provocative question and the candidate handled it extremely well. She made some powerful points in her answer and this impressed the panel.

POINTS FOR REFLECTION

- Have you spoken to peers who have recently been through the interview process?
- What questions were they asked?
- How did they answer?
- How would you respond?

STRUCTURED INTERVIEWS FOR SPECIALTY TRAINING POSTS

chapter 12

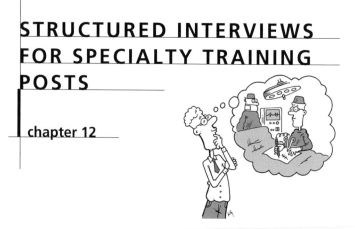

Specialty Training (ST1-6) structured interviews have certain characteristics that mean they are different from the interviews which used to be experienced at FY1 and FY2 levels, before these interviews largely disappeared with the arrival of computer-based 'matching programmes'. These, more senior, registrar level interviews usually involve at least 30 minutes direct contact time with panellists drawn from the relevant specialty. The questions posed at interview are usually based on the relevant person specification and application forms. Questions tend to be the same for all candidates, which means that panel members may struggle to separate one candidate from the next in their minds. Candidates' responses are usually marked according to a previously agreed scoring framework which links directly to the person specification. Rarely, candidates may face a single interview with a single panel, but the majority of specialties now tend to divide up the interview into

Getting that Medical Job: Secrets for Success, 3rd edition. © Colin J. Mumford and Suvankar Pal. Published 2011 by Blackwell Publishing Ltd.

10–15 minute themed 'stations' each assessed by a small group of independent panel members.

In general, these stations comprise a mixture of the following:

- 'Portfolio/CV' station
- 'Clinical scenario' station
- 'Ethical scenario' station
- 'Practical skills' station
- 'Research, audit and teaching' station
- 'Clinical governance and NHS Management' station

Each candidate's performance will be scored according to pre-determined criteria, with the individual stations being marked independently, before marks are summated to provide an overall score. This means that candidates can then be ranked in order of performance. Positions are offered to the highest ranked candidates with the next tranche being held 'in reserve' should offers to the highest placed candidates be declined.

GENERAL TIPS FOR THE DAY

Remember that being shortlisted for a specialty interview is quite an achievement in itself. Your fellow candidates may seem a little pleased with themselves, and you mustn't let the bravado of other candidates in the waiting room scare you off; they will be just as nervous as you are. As you enter the room for the start of each station take a deep breath, forget your performance at the previous station, smile and shake hands with the panel. And, as for any interview, you should try to relax, enjoy yourself and sound confident! The usual rules regarding body language and voice apply: maintain eye contact with all of the members of the panel, not just the person asking the questions. Remember to be enthusiastic and promote yourself as someone who as a colleague will contribute to the position in terms of expertise, enthusiasm, morale, energy, research, teaching, administration and make it abundantly clear that you really want the job!

If you are asked a challenging question, pause and reflect. Avoid saying the first thing that comes into your mind and at all costs avoid being confrontational unless you are particularly confident of your ground. If you're struggling to find an answer, for example to a clinical or ethical scenario, it is ok to say:

'That's quite a difficult question, but in practical terms what I would do in this situation is ...'

'... I would also seek advice from my colleagues and seniors, consult with the multidisciplinary team and be guided by local trust and national association guidelines ....'

Don't forget that you are a trainee working as part of a multidisciplinary team and you are not expected to know the answers to every question or have the means to cope with every given scenario.

Demonstrate reflective thinking when answering questions by drawing analogies with similar past experiences in your previous posts. Try to say things that will make you stand out from rival candidates in a positive way.

For example:

'You've given me a very challenging scenario. The way in which I have dealt with similar situations in the past, for example, includes....'

Whilst it is encouraged to have an opinion on ethical and governance issues, always deliver balanced arguments in response to questions, again drawing on your own experiences and avoid appearing dogmatic in your personal point of view.

For example:

'There are arguments both for and against enteral feeding in end-stage neurological disease and each patient's case needs to be evaluated individually. The issues I would consider include the wishes of the patient (after making an assessment of their capacity), their family and wider caregivers, the overall prognosis of their disease, any risks of the procedure itself, the patient's co-morbid medical conditions and

whether enteral feeding could be supported in the community. I would be cautious to advise that risks of aspiration inevitably persist despite enteral feeding and would probably point out that large clinical studies have demonstrated little benefit in terms of longer term survival and unclear effects on quality of life. However, I would need to research this in more detail by consulting local and national guidelines before providing the patient and their family with as much verbal and written information as possible. I would also consult with the nursing staff, speech and language therapists, and dieticians looking after the patient, perhaps also seeking an opinion from the gastroenterology nurse specialist who may be able to counsel the patient further. Ultimately, our role will be to work together as a team in providing sufficient information for the patient and their caregivers to make an informed choice.'

'PORTFOLIO/CV' STATION

In this station, the interview panel will systematically go through your portfolio of training, sometimes together with your application form and curriculum vitae. It is imperative that you spend time preparing your portfolio in detail with evidence of training achievements and work-based assessments completed in full. Make sure you 'know yourself' well! This is likely to be one of your chances to shine.

Potential questions

- Which of your workplace assessments (mini-CEX, DOPs, CBDs, MSFs, etc.) have been the most useful?
- Do you think personal development plans are important?
- Tell us about any academic prizes you have been awarded.
- Why did you undertake an intercalated BSc?
- Why did you choose the subject you did?
- Have you completed any parts of the MRCP/MRCS/MRCOG, etc.?

- You've done Part 1 – how do you think it went?
- Where do you see yourself in 5 years' time?
- How do you maintain your knowledge and skills as a medical trainee?
- Tell us about a recent situation you found stressful at work.
- What is your proudest achievement in medicine?
- What extracurricular interests do you have?
- What is your proudest achievement outside of medicine? Why does this help you to be a better doctor?
- Why should we employ you?
- What are your main strengths?
- What is your main weakness? (But see the comments in Chapter 10 on 'cringe questions' for advice on how to deal with this one.)
- If you walked onto a bus and found two friends talking about you, what would they be likely to be saying?

During this station, candidates are also often probed regarding their commitment and suitability for the specialty:

- Why have you chosen this specialty?
- Why in this particular region?
- Tell us about some recent courses you have attended.
- Why do you think you are particularly suited to this job?
- Are there any particular experiences you have had in your training which have contributed to your interest in this specialty?
- What have you done to assess this specialty as your career choice?
- Why do you think you are particularly suited to this specialty?
- What other specialties have you considered and why?

In general, the best answers for these questions draw on previous posts, personal acute on-call experience, outpatient experience, postgraduate meetings, courses and conferences, taster sessions and shadowing, research, audit, voluntary work and teaching.

- **What are the drawbacks of this specialty?**
- **Tell me about current research and advances in this specialty?**
- **What do you think about subspecialisation in this specialty?**
- **What are the biggest challenges facing this specialty over the next 10 years?**
- **Which regulatory bodies are involved in this specialty?**
- **Why Medicine and not General Practice?**
- **If you had to describe to your friends and family why you are choosing this specialty, what would you say?**

'CLINICAL AND ETHICAL SCENARIO' STATION

Scenarios in this station usually relate to emergencies or situations which may pose an ethical dilemma. Be familiar with the common emergencies relating to your chosen specialty.

Example of clinical scenarios

You have been called to assess a patient with known type 1 diabetes who has presented to A&E with a severe hypoglycaemic episode. How would you approach this situation?

Candidates are expected to provide a succinct account of emergency assessment and management including gathering a collateral history, rapid assessment of airway, breathing, circulation and conscious level followed by reversal of hypoglycaemia. The best candidates acknowledge when they would need input from senior colleagues or the critical care team and, eventually, the need to explore issues which have contributed to the patient's presentation such as poor compliance with treatment plans, and future implications for work and driving.

For some scenarios, the interview panel will progressively introduce new clinical material depending on a candidate's answers:

A 24-year-old lady is referred with headache and reduced conscious level. She has a background of rheumatoid arthritis and is taking methotrexate. Her GP has given intravenous benzylpenicillin. Discuss your management.

They might continue:

Her airway, breathing and circulation are stable. She is rousable but obtunded with no focal neurological signs. No senior colleagues are available. What would you do now?

The best candidates will recognise the likelihood of opportunistic infection in an immunosuppressed patient. Differential diagnoses would include bacterial or viral meningitis or encephalitis, toxic or metabolic disorders (relating to drugs, overdose, alcohol poisoning and so on). Candidates should discuss the need for a collateral history, the importance of a detailed general systemic examination, regular general and neurological observations and investigations including routine blood tests and cultures, followed by CT of the head – probably with anaesthetic cover – followed by a lumbar puncture.

The panel might go on with:

CSF studies demonstrate a lymphocytosis with a raised protein and low glucose. Does this suggest any particular organism? What treatment would you start?

A good answer would address the need for broad-spectrum antibiotics including benzylpencillin and a third generation cephalosporin (to cover Streptococcal infection and *Neisseria meningitis*), ampicillin to cover *Listeria* and aciclovir to treat potential viral encephalitis.

The next question might be:

Who else would you contact now?

A suitable answer would be the infectious diseases and critical care teams.

As this scenario continues, the panel will probe further, for example:

The patient develops seizures and has a further deterioration in conscious level. What would you do now?

The answer might state: re-examine the patient looking for signs of focal deficit, repeat neuroimaging and re-contact seniors with this new information. Consider the need for starting anticonvulsant medication.

Alternative scenarios might be:

- **How would you manage an 18-year-old patient with acute severe asthma presenting to A&E?**
- **An 85-year-old man presents with back pain following a fall and lower limb weakness. He has a past history of prostate cancer and is taking goserelin. What is the most likely cause? Why do you think this? What would you do?**
- **You chase routine bloods on a patient and find markedly raised urea and creatinine with a potassium of 6.8 mmol/L. What would you do next?**
- **A 28-year-old female is brought into A&E by paramedics unconscious. As the medical ST on call, you are bleeped down to resus.**
  What do you want to know over the phone?
  What would you do?
- **A 48-year-old female presents with pleuritic chest pain. She has a past history of a deep vein thrombosis. Discuss your approach.**

Example of ethics and communication skills scenarios

Many candidates are uneasy about dealing with ethical scenarios. Authors have written many texts over the years, and at least a passing knowledge of what these experts have said can be helpful. For example, Beauchamp and Childress set out the so-called 'four pillars of medical ethics'. These were:

- Non-maleficence (i.e. do no harm)
- Beneficence (act in the patient's best interests)
- Autonomy (respect the patient)
- Justice (aim for an equitable distribution of resources)

In general, the key point to get across is the importance of doing no harm to the patient, which should override all other ethical concerns. Acting in the best interest of the patient is clearly also crucial, and should feature in an answer to any question posed at interview, but be careful not to sound overly paternalistic when discussing this. 'Autonomy' relates to respect for the patient and serves as the basis for several ethical rules including informed consent, which could also be brought into an answer. Finally, you might recognise that medical resource is often scarce, and this may result in difficult choices for clinicians.

An example of a difficult ethical scenario that might be posed would be:

A 38-year-old lady with learning disability presents with symptoms suggestive of oesophageal varices. Following your assessment you feel an endoscopy is indicated but she is not happy to provide consent for this. Her mother is present.
What are your options for proceeding? How would you approach any ethical scenario like this one?

The best candidates would focus discussion on acting in the patient's best interest, discussing issues of capacity, consent and assent. They might mention the 'Adults with Incapacity Act', and show an awareness of the need to seek opinions from other members of the multidisciplinary team and also clearly identify other sources of advice including senior colleagues and professional bodies.

Other scenarios might be:

A patient with advanced dementia presents following a stroke. His swallow is unsafe and his son would like him to have a PEG inserted. The multidisciplinary team feel this is inappropriate.

What would you do?

How do you assess capacity?

What do you know about the Adults with Incapacity Act?

Whom can you ask for advice in this scenario?

Have you been in similar situations before?

Should patients generally have intravenous fluids withdrawn in this setting?

Have you come across a patient whom you felt should have had supportive treatments withdrawn but didn't?

How would you approach a confused patient with a recent upper GI bleed who is refusing an endoscopy?

You have been called to A&E by the FY2 on call to assess a 32-year-old lady who has just taken a paracetamol overdose. She is refusing admission. How would you approach this situation?

How would you manage an angry and anxious patient whom you recently diagnosed with epilepsy based on a detailed history and appropriate investigation results, and who has now gone home and read about sudden death in epilepsy? She has returned to the outpatient clinic without an appointment and is demanding to speak to you immediately about her worries.

Role-play

Some specialties, such as General Practice, use role-play for the assessment of clinical and ethical scenarios. When this happens, the role of the patient is generally played by a trained actor. These stations are designed to test communication skills and are similar to the examination technique used in the MRCP PACES examination. Candidates may be asked to take a history or provide information and counselling. Rather than assessing clinical knowledge, the emphasis of these stations is on building rapport with patients, demonstrating effective skills in listening and empathy, and communicating complex concepts in lay terms avoiding the use of medical jargon.

Communication skills

Inevitably an interview panel will want to satisfy themselves that you have decent communication skills. Potential questions would include the following:

Give an example of how you won the trust of a worried and sceptical patient.
Described what you did and why?
What effect did it have on both you and the patient?

Very good answers would demonstrate the following:
- Responding to needs and concerns with interest and understanding
- Acting in an open, non-judgmental manner
- Attempting to generate a safe and trusting atmosphere
- Making efforts to understand patient concerns
- Reassuring the patient with appropriate words and actions

Other instructions from the panel might be:

Please describe a time when you have needed to explain a complicated procedure or medical term to a patient.
How did you do this?
What was the outcome?

Here, good answers would demonstrate the following:
- Adjusting the style of questioning/response as appropriate

- An ability to express ideas clearly to others
- Clarity in both verbal and written communication
- Flexibility in style to suit recipient
- Tailoring communication and establishing a relationship of respect with others

THE 'PRACTICAL SKILLS' STATION

This type of station is more common in surgical specialties, anaesthetics and obstetrics and gynaecology. Candidates may be asked to demonstrate practical skills such as suturing or asked to perform procedures on manikins, for example intubation. In some surgical specialties, manual dexterity is assessed using hand held laparoscopic kits.

Other practical stations could include the following:
- **Assessment of medical note taking:** Candidates may be shown a video clip of a consultant assessing a patient on a ward round. They are then asked to record a ward round entry on continuation sheets.
- **Prescribing station:** Candidates might be presented with a clinical vignette, then asked to check a patient's drug chart looking for any prescribing errors or omissions.

'RESEARCH, AUDIT AND TEACHING'

Questions that might arise in this station would be:

Is it important for doctors to do research?
Why have you done research? Should we all do it? If so, is that feasible?
Is pursuing a higher degree (MD/PhD) desirable? Why?

The best answers to these questions would focus on the following issues:
- The fact that research is crucial for advancing medical knowledge, encouraging curiosity, providing greater understanding

of underlying pathophysiological mechanisms of disease and ultimately informing best clinical practice.

- All doctors need to be able to evaluate original research in order to inform their own practice.
- A formal period in research allows doctors to gain insight into research and statistical methodologies and a deeper understanding of critically appraising literature.
- Research also fosters generic skills of persistence, inquisitiveness, an ability to think laterally and an ability to work to deadlines and under pressure.
- By immersing interest in one area it may also encourage the development of a subspecialty interest in the future.

Should research be mandatory for all doctors?
Is there a role for specialist MSc courses and diplomas?

If you have done research, then it will certainly be asked about. For example:

- **Which of your publications is in the journal with the highest impact factor? What was your role in writing that paper?**
- **What factors make research in this specialty particularly challenging?**
- **What is your understanding of the concept of 'evidence-based' medicine?**
- **What are the pros and cons of evidence-based practice?**
- **What are the different levels of evidence available?**
- **Tell us about the last paper you read that changed your practice.**
- **How would you design a study to answer the question about how best to treat condition x?**

Critical appraisal of a research paper

In some interviews, candidates are given a few minutes to evaluate an original research paper. Interviewers then may ask questions relating to the study design, research methodologies, data interpretation, the statistical methods used for data analysis, and discussion of findings.

Audit increasingly features in interview questions

Candidates might be asked:

Is clinical audit important? Why?
Discuss audits you have been involved with.
What was your specific role?
What were the significant results?
What do you understand about the audit cycle?
Have you ever completed the audit loop?
If you were to do an audit in your current job, what would you do it on?

Teaching is likely to be considered

For example:

Tell us about your teaching experience.
Have you been on any teaching courses?
Do you think formal teaching qualifications are important?
What methods of teaching are you familiar with? Which do you prefer and why?
Have you taught disciplines other than medicine? What was different in your delivery?

'CLINICAL GOVERNANCE AND NHS MANAGEMENT'

Candidates must ensure that they are aware of current issues affecting the profession as a whole as well as specific issues relating to their chosen specialty. A clear grasp of news reported in the medical press such as '*BMJ News*' and '*Hospital Doctor*' would be a good starting point. There are a number of generic topics you will be expected to be aware of, and the panel will expect you to have formulated an opinion. For example:

What do you think about the following:
- **Modernising medical careers**
- **The European working time directive**
- **Hospital at night**
- **The role of clinical nurse specialists and advanced nurse practitioners**
- **The merger of the General Medical Council (GMC) and the Postgraduate Medical Education and Training Board (PMETB) and the thinking and planning behind that merger**
- **Revalidation and re-certification**
- **New methods of delivering clinical services and how things can be improved including managed clinical networks and community health partnerships**
- **Improving patient choice, e.g. the 'choose and book' system for making outpatient appointments, market-style incentives, multiple providers, national targets to improve performance such as reducing waiting times (in A&E, for outpatient appointments, for suspected cancer referrals)**
- **Costs associated with introducing new drugs and technologies**
- **How service delivery may have to change depending on financial climates**

What do you know about Clinical Governance?
How does Clinical Governance affect patient safety?
How does Clinical Governance impact on your daily work?
Who, in your hospital, is responsible for Clinical Governance?
What is Clinical Risk Management?

Other questions in this station might include the following:
With others taking over the work of doctors how do you make sure that you are being adequately trained?

How would you manage poor performance in your team?

How would you manage misconduct?

What is the difference between management and leadership?

How would you manage conflict in the workplace?

What is your understanding of equality and diversity in the workplace?

How do you manage paperwork?

How do you organise your day?

What are the attributes of a good team player?

Give us a recent example of a time where you worked as a member of a multidisciplinary team.

What leadership skills have you acquired during your training?

Have you ever been in a situation where you have had a conflict with a colleague?

Describe a time when pressure at work has called you to feel upset or angry:
- What was the cause of you feeling pressured?
- What did you do?
- What was the outcome?

Tell us what you understand about the GMC's 'Duties of a Doctor' guide.

People organise their time in different ways. What approaches and strategies do you use to plan/protect your time for training?

How do you prioritise conflicting demands?

How do you justify your actions?

What is important?

The best answers would incorporate the following points:
- Thinking ahead, preparing and planning effectively
- Coordinating activities appropriately
- Building contingencies to deal with shifting demands

- Understanding limitations, constraints and working within them
- Prioritising conflicting demands
- Juggling competing demands

Have you ever been angry or frustrated with a patient? Discuss the background to this. How did you feel? What did you do? Did you speak to anyone? What did they advise? If your FY1 had similar issues, how would you tackle it and what advice would you give?

Hospital administrators and lay members of the panel may well ask about safety, governance and risk. For example:

What is an adverse incident? What is a near miss?
Have you ever been involved in a critical incident?
What happened? Outcome? Did you write an incident form? What was the outcome of that form? Has it affected departmental practice?

Tell us about a clinical mistake you have made. What was the situation? Did you complete a significant event analysis on it?

Describe a time when you had to tell a patient that a mistake had been made, either by you or someone else.
- **What did you say?**
- **How did you justify your actions?**
- **How did it affect your work afterwards?**

Strong responses to these questions would focus on the following:
- Demonstrating respect for patients and colleagues
- Being positive when dealing with problems
- Awareness of the need to learn from mistakes
- Being committed to equality of care for all
- Putting patients' needs before your own when appropriate

- Backing own judgement appropriately
- Attempting to learn from incident to avoid future similar episodes
- Adverse incident monitoring including appropriate documentation and learning from critical incident and near misses
- Risk control (record keeping and documentation)
- Rapid response to complaints

Handling problem colleagues

How would you handle a problem colleague? Examples are:

- **Substance misuse in a colleague**
- **A colleague who is continuously late/poor at attending handover**
- **A colleague who consistently makes bad clinical judgements and mistakes.**

The best responses to these questions would acknowledge the duty of care to patients, an obligation to the multiprofessional team, the duty of care to the troubled colleague, and duty to the NHS Trust (i.e. to the employer). With regard to substance abuse, for example, the doctor in question should be removed from the workplace. It would be imperative to ensure that no harm has come to patients who have been in contact with this doctor. This might involve reviewing all clinical decisions made, including any drugs prescribed or interventions undertaken. All clinical duties which would have been taken by the doctor in question would need to be adequately covered. Duty of care to the troubled doctor would include maintaining confidence and exploring the reasons behind the substance misuse. Clearly, any dangerous behaviour would need to be reported to the supervising consultant, educational supervisor and postgraduate dean.

POINTS FOR REFLECTION

- How would you answer the interview questions detailed in this chapter?
- Practise your answers with friends, family, peers and senior colleagues.

THE ACADEMIC INTERVIEW AND INTERVIEWS FOR CLINICAL RESEARCH FELLOWSHIPS

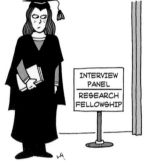

chapter 13

With the arrival of run-through training, the requirement to undertake a formal period of research before entering higher specialist training has diminished. Nevertheless, many medical graduates wish to spend a period of time devoted to work leading to a higher research degree, often with a view to developing a career in academic medicine, or fostering a subspecialty interest. Doctorate degrees include the Doctor of Medicine (MD) and Doctor of Philosophy (PhD, DPhil or equivalent). These degrees, examined following submission of a thesis, promote and assess original, independent and critical thinking and encourage the ability to develop and understand theoretical concepts. A period of research may be clinical or laboratory based, and inevitably will encourage the development of ability to recognise and analyse problems, gaining of knowledge of recent advances within the relevant field and related areas, promote an understanding of research methodologies and techniques, and generate an understanding of their appropriate application within

Getting that Medical Job: Secrets for Success, 3rd edition. © Colin J. Mumford and Suvankar Pal. Published 2011 by Blackwell Publishing Ltd.

the research field. Individuals who spend time in research also gain the ability critically to analyse and evaluate the research findings of others, and an ability to summarise, document, report and reflect on progress of their own work, and that of co-workers in the field.

Research studentships may be advertised with funding allocated for pre-specified projects, or alternatively, would-be researchers may apply for independent clinical research fellowships or academic training programmes. It is vital that you thoroughly research the fellowship you are applying for (including looking closely at the funding available, for example does this include any fees and the cost of consumables?). Application rounds for clinical research fellowships funded by bodies such as the Medical Research Council (MRC) and Wellcome Foundation Application typically take place twice per year. Applicants are shortlisted following peer review of their research proposal, and are then invited to a panel interview. If successful, it may easily take a year from submission of an application to the point at which an award is granted, and the resulting research can begin.

Applications for any such research post must be completed clearly and economically with a well-defined case for support, presentation of a detailed and focused hypothesis, and give a clear justification for why you want to perform this research. A robust study design must be clearly outlined including a statement of proposed statistical methodology, and – if relevant – a power calculation to permit determination of the necessary sample size. The application form must fully justify all the funding for which you are competing. Proposals for research projects which appear to be unfocused, unoriginal or overambitious are likely to be rejected. In addition, there must be a clear training element. The centre in which research is to be undertaken must generally be of high standing and the applicant must demonstrate that they have the potential capacity to develop into a competitive researcher.

The research interview is often led by a carefully put-together panel made of a number of experts in the proposed field, who will collect evidence regarding the merits of the proposed research, and who will score the proposal against key pre-defined criteria. Questioning will be shared by the various panel members who will record their own private scores. There will then be discussion and a review of final rankings. In addition to questions relating to personal attributes, candidates should inevitably expect more detailed questions relating to wider issues of research and academia. Potential topics for the research interview might include, 'personal research experience', 'The Clinical Research Fellowship', 'research interest and motivation', and discussion surrounding 'understanding of academic medicine'.

EXAMPLES OF QUESTIONS RELATING TO PERSONAL RESEARCH EXPERIENCE

Tell us about your undergraduate thesis.

- **Highlight your personal contribution to the project.**
- **Discuss the experimental design, statistical analysis and any resulting publications.**

Tell us about other research you have carried out.

- **What difficulties did you experience?**
- **How did you overcome these?**
- **If you did it again, what would you do differently?**

In answering questions like these, be prepared to discuss case reports and publications and presentations that you have been involved in as a medical student and junior doctor. Specifically, you should say what your personal involvement in the study design was, how you obtained ethical approval, your processes for data collection, data analysis and how you approached writing up the work. Do not worry about any lack of publications; these will come later and interview panels are not usually perturbed by few or even no publications if you are in the early stages of your career.

Other areas for discussion might include:

> **Discuss clinical implications of research you've done.**
>
> **Talk about ethical considerations in setting up your research.**
>
> **Outline a piece of research that you have been involved in, with particular reference to aims, objectives, methodology, evaluation, limitations or improvements. How would you link your objective to the final evaluation?**
>
> **Tell about research that you've been involved with, as if you were talking to a layperson. What were its overall implications?**

Having a clear answer to the latter question is particularly important. Panels place great weight on the ability of a candidate to be able to present future research in a clear and concise manner, with plain language, and avoiding too much jargon or technical terminology. If some small piece of work has already been done, then it is imperative that you are able to say what question you asked at the start of the research, what answer you obtained, and what the significance of that finding was. Remember that not everyone on the panel will know the field that you are describing, and you must be able to 'set the scene' by explaining the rationale behind your previous research, and be able to speak about it in simple terms.

THE CLINICAL RESEARCH FELLOWSHIPS

For more senior research positions such as these, you will need to have done your groundwork very thoroughly indeed. Get 'mock interviews' from senior academics in your present workplace before you attend the interview. Be ready to address all of the following points in some detail:

Why this specific project?
Why do you want to work at this institution?

You should ensure that you have done enough research to answer these questions with considerable precision. Nothing should be, or appear to be, 'half-hearted'. You need to have considered all the details, including diverse aspects like facilities, people, links between hospital and the laboratory, and future plans to develop the research further if it goes well.

What motivated/inspired you to get involved in research in this topic?

Have an answer ready, for example you might refer to a particular patient you've looked after, an audit project you've been involved in, or discuss relevant research papers you have read.

What attracts you to this particular academic scheme?
What are the disadvantages of this particular academic scheme?

For Academic Clinical Fellowships, you do not need to be too specific about your current research interests, because one of the purposes of most academic schemes is to allow you to explore and to develop your interests during the first 1 or 2 years. It is more important to demonstrate an understanding of, enthusiasm for, and commitment to, an academic career.

Personal research interest and motivation

You need to be prepared to explain why you want to spend time in a period of research, especially bearing in mind that many postgraduate tutors no longer consider it necessary, and indeed some postgraduate deans are being told to *discourage* research, since it delays the production of 'fully-trained' specialists. So you should be prepared to answer any of these questions:

Talk briefly about a paper that you have read recently that interested you. Why did it appeal?

Tell us about a recent research article that you have read and critically evaluate it.

What papers have you read that have changed your clinical practice recently?

What clinical problems have you encountered that you would like to solve?

If you had unlimited research funding, what is the question that you would most like to address and how would you do so?

What attracts you to your chosen specialty?

Why would you like to pursue a MD rather than a PhD (or vice versa)?

Where do you see yourself in 10 years' time?

What do you bring to an academic career and what do you need now from an academic scheme?

What will you do if you are not successful in the application for this post?

Understanding of academic medicine

You are likely to need to justify your self-belief that you can become a decent researcher, and that you appreciate some of the challenges involved. So be ready to deal with these:

Is it possible to combine research and clinical work (and teaching)?

How will your choice of an academic career impact on your clinical training?

• **What steps will you take in this regard?**

What do you understand by the term 'translational medicine'?

Do medical clinicians make good scientists?

What are the qualities of a good researcher?

Are animal experiments important? Can you give me any examples?

Tell me about the use of good-quality controls in experiments?

How do you evaluate the quality of evidence presented in a study?

What do you understand about case control studies, cohort studies, randomised-controlled double blind trials, meta-analyses of trials?

What do you understand by clinical and research governance?

What ethical considerations do you think may be important in this research project?

How would you explain this research project to a lay member of public?

Should funding for medical research be prioritised over spending for existing patients?

How will the credit crunch affect funding of medical research?

IMPORTANT POINTS REGARDING THE CONSULTANT INTERVIEW

chapter 14

Most of the preceding sections of this book have been concerned with the generality of medical job interviews for all grades of post. Much of what we have written is relevant not just to junior-level appointments but also to those at senior level. However, it is worth spending some time considering specific points that are only really relevant to an interview for a consultant grade post.

The most obvious differences between interviews for junior medical posts and interviews for posts at consultant level are first, the size of the interview panel, and secondly, the length of the interview. In a consultant interview it is likely that there will be as many as twelve people present around the interview table. It is a running certainty that there will be a combination of consultant medical staff, managers and administrators present. There may well also be the lay representative referred to earlier. The second point is that consultant interviews are often much more of a discursive two-way process, i.e. passing around a wide range of topics, with a discussion between equals, in which the panel are genuinely interested in the opinions of

Getting that Medical Job: Secrets for Success, 3rd edition. © Colin J. Mumford and Suvankar Pal. Published 2011 by Blackwell Publishing Ltd.

the various candidates, with scope for mutual education and sometimes disagreement between panel and candidate, without this necessarily being a problem or detriment to appointment. Hence, many of these interviews can extend to 45 minutes or even longer.

The other key point to stress is that as a candidate you need to be sensitive to what the interview panel is looking for. *This may be slightly different from what you expect:* in contrast to junior-level interviews where the emphasis may be on obtaining the very best candidate in terms of academic brilliance, the emphasis in appointing a consultant colleague is often not so demanding in terms of intellectual excellence. Obviously, the panel is concerned to make sure they appoint an individual who is entirely capable of doing the job in question, but they realise also that they are appointing a candidate whom they may be working with for more than 30 years. Therefore, it is essential that they find somebody who is not just a 'safe pair of hands', but also someone whom they can be pretty certain that they will get on with in years to come. This means that personality, warmth and affability, backed up by secure professionalism, may well win over a panel in preference to the cold candidate who simply radiates academic supremacy.

Some aspects of the interview will, of course, be similar to more junior-level appointments. Inevitably there will be a review of your curriculum vitae to make sure that your training has been fully completed and that you are at the stage where you're eligible for appointment to a consultant post. Once that is established, however, it is likely that the panel will seek to establish what specifically you would bring to the department if you were appointed; for example, would you bring experience of new anaesthetic techniques, new surgical skills, or some other new specialist knowledge to enhance the existing abilities and skills of the department. In addition, your potential future colleagues will probably also be keen to know if they will be able to shed some of their own administrative load, perhaps by establishing whether you would take on responsibility for organising undergraduate or postgraduate teaching, perhaps seeing if you would be willing to take on the management of the weekly departmental meetings and so on.

Remember also that in an interview at this level, the panel does not want bland uninspiring answers to the questions that they pose. Some sort of discussion and controversy is entirely reasonable. For example, maybe there has been recent publication of a high-profile academic paper describing a new technique for monitoring a certain illness with which you work, but you feel that the paper was flawed in terms of its methodology, or the conclusions drawn. If so, this sort of thing may provide a useful basis for discussion and crosstalk in the interview. Equally, if one of the non-medical members of the panel asks somewhat banal or cringeworthy questions, for example bringing up the nightmare of 'strengths and weaknesses', (described as 'googlies' in a previous chapter of this book), then from time to time a very aggressive answer may bear fruit. For example, one of the authors of this book was made aware of an individual being appointed to the board of a major British pharmaceutical company. This was an extremely high-level appointment and all the candidates were very senior in their field. One candidate was asked (by an external member of the panel) '...and what are your weaknesses?' After a short pause, he replied: 'Well, I have to confess that at times I do find myself answering bloody stupid questions in senior-level interviews.' This was an example of a robust, aggressive answer, and was a comment which was highly unorthodox and therefore would be dangerous in a junior-level interview. But in this extremely senior situation it was probably a reasonable response to give, and certainly would have made the other members of the interview panel sit up and pay more attention to what was going on. The candidate was successful.

Another example of a robust controversial answer to a question posed in a consultant-level interview related to audit. The candidate was asked to explain to the panel what they thought about the increasing use of 'audit' in local hospitals. The answer that came was a well considered explanation that in the candidate's opinion audit was a word used simply as a euphemism for poor quality clinical research which was not subject to the rigorous process of peer review and which could never be published in the medical journals. In the candidate's opinion audit should be abolished, and replaced by high quality, relevant clinical research, and therefore no hospital should continue to be involved with audit. This was a perfect example of an answer that would be catastrophic in an interview at registrar level. However, in the environment of a senior-level consultant post interview it seemed to be an entirely reasonable answer and resulted in many members of the panel nodding their heads vigorously in approval at what had just been said.

In the financially-aware health service of the 21st century, you may also find yourself being asked about matters such as the proposed job plan in the consultant interview.

You will inevitably have seen the job plan outline, since it should have been sent to you with the basic details of the post, and you should know, in advance of the interview, how intense the weekly workload that is proposed is going to be. You may also be invited to comment on the proposed split between 'direct clinical care' programmed activities and so-called 'supporting professional activities' in the job plan. In the opinion of the authors the interview itself is not the ideal forum in which to start negotiation relating to the precise structure of the job that you will take up if successful. Nevertheless, if these areas are brought up in the interview then it would be entirely reasonable to point out that based on what you have seen so far the proposed job plan is either too heavy, unworkable, or conceivably 'rather too light' for you, bearing in mind your aspirations for what you hope to bring to the department.

Salaries should not be discussed at all during the interview. Rather you should save that sort of delicate negotiation for the period of time once the interview is completed, as described in a subsequent section of this book. So if the question of remuneration is brought up by a member of the panel, our advice would be to acknowledge the question, but politely point out that – if offered the post – you would 'look forward to addressing this and related issues with the chief executive and financial director of the hospital in the fullness of time'. Often nowadays there is very little scope to negotiate the starting salary, but it may be worth trying. More about this subject later.

EXPLAINING TIME-OUT FROM TRAINING

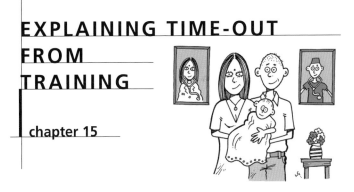

chapter 15

CAREER GAPS TO HAVE CHILDREN

Like it or not, there can be specific problems that some candidates, especially women, will face in a medical job interview. Historically, hospital consultants have tended to be male and often quite conservative in their outlook. Most members—and certainly the chairman—of an interview panel are now acutely aware that there are significant restrictions on the the type of questions that can be asked of a female candidate, and all would agree that questions such as, 'Are you thinking of leaving six months after appointment to have children?' are both unacceptable and outrageous. Nevertheless, the fact that your curriculum vitae shows that you have already had a year or two off in order to have children may, no matter how inappropriately, be brought up during the interview. And this problem is no longer confined to females, since many male interview candidates have now taken periods of time off work as 'extended paternity leave' or similar.

Getting that Medical Job: Secrets for Success, 3rd edition. © Colin J. Mumford and Suvankar Pal. Published 2011 by Blackwell Publishing Ltd.

With a little forethought, troublesome questions like these can be turned to your advantage. It is entirely reasonable to explain to an interview panel that your two main priorities in life are, first, your family and, secondly, your career. And stress to the panel that the priorities *go in that order*. Most interview panels would have to agree that there is 'never a right time' in the ascent of the hospital doctor career ladder to have children, and the majority will be impressed by someone who has managed to juggle pregnancy, babies, young children and a career as a junior hospital doctor.

You may be able to make light of an inappropriate question and 'spin' the answer to your advantage. For example, you might comment that you have benefited from experience of sleepless nights and now have 'great experience in dealing with vomiting'. You could observe that unlike other members of the panel you have now—perhaps—been a patient yourself and have come to realise what it is like waiting a prolonged period of time for an outpatient appointment, or worse still waiting several hours before an anaesthetist came to give you an epidural. You might move on to say that your experience as a pregnant mother – or a new father – has given you rare insights into some of the more irritating aspects of hospital practice such as being dealt with by doctors and nurses who fail to introduce themselves.

In general terms, even the most fuddy-duddy consultants on an interview panel now realise that the 'work–life balance' is important, and they will respect somebody who is able to talk about it authoritatively during a formal interview. So the main message here is: if the panel tries to attack you with an inappropriate or outrageous question make sure that you 'come out fighting' and hit back hard at them.

APPLYING FOR A JOB SHARE

The concept of the 'job share' is not new. In many walks of life, particularly in industry and the Civil Service, job sharing is now commonplace. Unfortunately, it is observed less frequently in day-to-day hospital practice. There is no good reason for this, and if you feel that the most appropriate next move on the career ladder is to a post that is shared with another individual then do not hesitate to apply for such a position. More importantly, be aware that a post that is advertised as a full-time job can often be performed highly effectively by two people job sharing, so be prepared to go and speak to the relevant consultants and human resources department to suggest that a full-time job which they have just advertised could perhaps be filled by means of a job share.

The key point that needs to be considered when applying for a job-share post in a hospital is whether to apply in the hope that another like-minded individual will also apply to make up the 'other half' of the job share, or whether you should apply with a 'ready-made partner' and present yourselves as a unit of two people in the interview. If at all possible, we would suggest that the latter approach is the better of the two. If you enter an interview seeking to work in a job-share post and make it plain that you're already on good terms with the other doctor applying, then you will be well placed to counter any anxieties on the part of the panel regarding logistics and communication between the two doctors who would fulfil a single role. A panel may, for example, ask what you would do if your child became ill during one of the days when you should be working in hospital. The fact that you knew your job-share partner in advance of the interview would then allow you to say that you had already made contingency plans for such eventualities. They may well ask how you would communicate about your patients, and you should explain that you would follow a standard professional 'hand over' procedure as used by all other doctors. Your goal must be to reassure the panel that you and your job-sharing partner would fill the post on offer with as much, if not greater, reliability than a single person.

OTHER DELAYS IN CAREER PROGRESS

There are a number of other reasons, again not necessarily specific to female candidates, for an apparent delay in an individual's career progression which may alarm members of an interview panel. Examples would include time taken off in order to look after elderly parents, time spent abroad accompanying a partner on a sabbatical or other overseas placement, and perhaps time spent doing a prolonged adventurous activity such as a year-long round-the-world yacht race. The art of dealing with these issues during a job interview is to make sure that you are not pushed into viewing these periods of time as any sort of a negative experience; rather you should present them as a positive experience which sets you apart from the other candidates. You will need to stress that although your medical career inevitably was put on hold as a result of these activities, you have gained in so many other ways, be they cultural, linguistic, or simply by gaining an in-depth experience of the 'receiving end' of the National Health Service.

WHAT HAPPENS BEHIND THE SCENES?

chapter 16

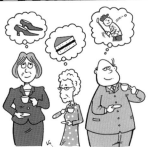

WHO CHOOSES THE PANEL AND HOW ARE PANEL MEMBERS SELECTED?

The composition of the interview panel will vary according to the grade of post for which you are applying. In years gone by, it was not unknown for old-style junior house officer (JHO) and stand-alone senior house officer (SHO) appointments to be made by a couple of consultants rather hastily grabbed on the day of the interview, or possibly asked if they were able to interview just the day before. This situation has now changed, and panels are usually (but not always) convened on a much more formal basis. Things are definitely more formalised for appointments to specialty training posts at registrar level, and are very much more rigid for appointments to consultant positions. For hospital training posts it is generally the local postgraduate medical department that will take responsibility for convening the panel. In contrast, if the appointment is for a consultant post then the hospital management will almost certainly take on

Getting that Medical Job: Secrets for Success, 3rd edition. © Colin J. Mumford and Suvankar Pal. Published 2011 by Blackwell Publishing Ltd.

that duty, and it will usually be the director of human resources or his deputy who is responsible for the selection of panel members.

In the earlier sections of this book, we mentioned the absolute requirement for certain individuals to be on the interview panel, particularly for appointments at specialist registrar and consultant level. These are the representatives of the relevant Royal Colleges, previously called 'national panellists' in Scotland. For each medical specialty in every part of the country there are often only a few individuals who are able to fulfil the role of Royal College representative and therefore the date of interview and the selection of the other members of the interview panel are often determined by the availability of that person. Personnel departments that are trying to set up an interview will usually contact the Royal College representative first and, once they have secured their availability for a specific date, then the other members of the panel are chosen. Usually, human resources departments find that they have relatively little choice in the availability of other consultants to act as members of an interview panel, because of clinical and teaching commitments as well as other engagements. However, for some posts, particularly at consultant level, there is a minimum number of individuals who are required to be on an interview panel in order for it to be 'quorate', and, accordingly, consultants may sometimes be plucked out of their clinical work to sit on a panel at very short notice indeed. As a result, the group of consultants who find their way onto an interview panel is often something of a random selection.

WHO IS THE CHAIRMAN?

The chairman of an interview panel—particularly for consultant grade appointments—is usually a senior consultant from a specialty which is *not* the one to which an appointment is being made. The main role of the chairman is to ensure 'fair play', and therefore there is some merit in that individual not being a close colleague of the other members of the panel, almost all of whom *will* be specialists in the relevant discipline. This rule does not hold true for very junior or locum appointments, when the chairman of the panel could simply be one of the assembled team of physicians or surgeons selected at the start of the interview by his colleagues. It is important to note that, strictly speaking, the chairman of the interview panel is a non-voting member, but this is variable between hospitals. They do, however, take responsibility for collating the votes of members of the panel at the end of the interview process, and in the event of a tie, they would almost certainly be obliged to make a 'casting vote'.

WHAT ARE THEY TOLD BEFOREHAND?

The interview panel will usually be asked to attend the interview room some 15–20 minutes before the arrival of the first candidate. If the chairman of the panel is good at his job, then a semi-formal briefing of the other panel members will take place. The chairman will ensure that all members of the panel have been introduced to each other and that they appreciate who is the Royal College representative. He will remind the panel members what the post is that they are about to appoint, he will instruct them that all discussion within the interview room is confidential and he will also ensure that none of the panel members has any 'conflict of interest' in the interview process. This latter point may present a problem in interviews for appointments to small specialties, for example if several local specialist registrars are applying for a consultant post in their own hospital. Under these circumstances, it is very probable that some of the local consultants may be on friendly terms with the specialist registrars and, if that is the case, there is a requirement—at least in theory—that panel members declare it. Such an announcement does not, however, preclude a consultant's ability to remain on the panel: the chairman will simply make note of what has been said and confirm with the remaining members of the panel that they do not consider it to be a problem.

In recent years, there has been one significant change in the instructions given to interview panel members, and many of them find this rather irritating. Namely, the chairman of the panel will advise them that they should address *the same question to each candidate* who is interviewed. The logic behind this new development is understandable, as it removes one potential variable in the interview process, and arguably leads to a fairer outcome. Unfortunately, most panel members do not like this instruction, since they would prefer to ask different questions according to the background and experience of the candidate whom they are interviewing, and often want to frame their questions in reaction to answers which have been given by the interviewee up to that point. Frustratingly, it is not possible to know in advance of your own interview whether you will receive exactly the same set of questions as all the candidates who have been interviewed before you, but this is now certainly a possibility.

WHAT DO THEY DISCUSS WHEN YOU'VE GONE?

When the final interview candidate has left the room, the chairman of the interview panel will usually look around, smile at his colleagues, and say: 'Right, who's for coffee?' There then follows five minutes of relaxed discussion, usually relating either to golf or to the most recent model of convertible Mercedes. This happy diversion is eventually brought to a close by the chairman who will attempt to 'bring the panel to order', and will remind the panel members that there is some 'work to do'.

The precise sequence of what happens next varies from panel to panel and is generally determined by the chairman. Typically, the chairman of the panel will turn to the Royal College representative and will ask whether all the candidates are suitable for appointment or not. It is very unusual for the Royal College representative to find that one or more individuals cannot be appointed for some reason, but should that be the case, then this is the point at which they will say so. The excluded candidate or candidates will not be considered any further during the selection process.

Once this particular formality is over, every other member of the interview panel will then be invited to say a few words about the various applicants. In general terms, most panel members will conclude their comments by suggesting their preferred 'one, two, three'. In other words, this is the stage during the interview process when each panel member makes a suggestion as to which candidate, they think, is the most appropriate, who is second best and who is third best. The chairman of the panel will take responsibility for collating these observations made by panel members. Usually, he will record these views on a formal 'voting grid', marking '1', '2', '3' and so on, alongside each candidate's name. Surprisingly, there is often broad agreement between panel members as to which are the three or four best candidates, and the same names are heard in each member's summary of their views. If this is the case, then the chairman simply looks at his grid and may be able to make an immediate announcement as to which is the successful candidate based on what he has heard so far, i.e. he can add up the numbers on the grid in front of him, and the candidate with the *lowest* score will be the first to be appointed, *provided that that candidate gained a vote from every panel member*. In the same way—if several appointments are being made, for example, to a number of specialist registrar posts—the chairman will be able to use the scoring grid in order to work out which candidate has come second, which third, up to the required number of appointees for the posts on offer.

Sometimes, the chairman will instruct the interview panel to consider the candidates in a different way. Rather than asking for votes, he may suggest that the panel has a general discussion, to see if there are any candidates who have just been interviewed who are clearly not going to be in the top three or four. Again, if there is agreement between the interview panel, then these names will be deleted and excluded from further discussion. This mechanism then leaves the panel with just three or four names to consider, and further discussion will then ensue with the chairman finally asking the panel to remove another one or two names, leaving final consideration of—perhaps—just the top two. There will then be a similar voting process, except all members of the panel will simply be asked to say who is their 'number one' and who is their 'number two'. In this way, a clear decision is usually reached.

Obviously, these systems are not universal, and often a different strategy is needed if a large number of posts are being appointed, for example to a large specialist registrar training rotation in a major teaching hospital, or if there are just two candidates for a senior professorship. Nevertheless, candidates can be reassured that enormous effort goes into making sure that the appointments process is as fair as it can be, and unsuccessful candidates who come away from interviews announcing that they consider the panel was 'rigged' or that the appointment was a 'set-up' are almost invariably wrong.

HOW IMPORTANT ARE THE REFERENCES?

Most interview candidates would be surprised to learn that the references play relatively little part in the interview process. Indeed, it is very often the case that references are not consulted until the panel has decided who are the top one or two candidates. Sometimes, the final decision is made with recourse to the references taking place only as an afterthought. The main role of the reference, therefore, is as an instrument to reassure the panel that the decision which they have made on the strength of the interview is the correct one.

It is not unheard of for the panel to decide who is their preferred first choice and who their second choice, and then find something slightly untoward or possibly disturbing in the reference for the winning candidate. Under these circumstances, the chairman will usually ask the panel if they wish to reconsider the order of their 'top two', and sometimes the individual who was positioned in second place is then awarded the job. Accordingly, having top-quality references is highly important, but your references may only play a crucial part right at the very end of the interview process.

AFTER THE INTERVIEW

chapter 17

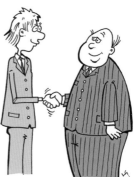

THE JOB OFFER

If all has gone according to plan then a short while after the interview is finished the chairman of the panel will come out of the interview room and will invite you to 'come back in'. Almost always—but not absolutely inevitably—this means that you are the successful candidate and effectively means that you have got the job. Resist the urge to start hugging your fellow candidates at this stage, most of whom will suddenly feel an intense dislike towards you. Smile sweetly and try to look sympathetically towards the other candidates before smiling in a professional manner at the chairman of the interview panel and re-entering the room.

You will be invited to sit down and the chairman of the panel will announce something along the lines of: 'We are delighted

Getting that Medical Job: Secrets for Success, 3rd edition. © Colin J. Mumford and Suvankar Pal. Published 2011 by Blackwell Publishing Ltd.

to be able to offer you the job.' Strictly speaking, the chairman of the interview panel has just made a significant error of protocol, since in fact interview panels do not 'offer jobs', they simply make recommendations to the management of the hospital or to the regional postgraduate dean regarding whom should be appointed. Only in exceptional circumstances, however, is the individual who is recommended by the interview panel not the person eventually selected for the job by the hospital. You should continue to retain a professional air and should thank the panel and agree that you will accept the job. A word of warning is necessary here since in the excitement of the moment it is very easy to make a mistake and announce that you will not just accept the job but readily also accept all the unsatisfactory aspects of the job which you read about in the job description but chose to ignore up until this point. You might be better placed to thank the interview panel and announce that you will, 'look forward to receiving their formal offer in the next day or two'. The reason why we advise a cagey approach at this point is that it is during the time between the interview and before formally accepting the offer of employment that you may need to negotiate certain aspects of the post. This tends to be far more important at consultant level than at specialist registrar level. You may now return home or, as is sometimes the case, accept an invitation go out for a beer with the interview panel, but whatever happens you can look forward to receiving a written letter offering you the job during the next few days.

NEGOTIATION

Negotiation at this stage may be all important. Remember that this is the first stage in the job application process at which you are in a position of power. You must not abuse that power since an aggressive negotiation style will go down very badly with your future colleagues, and the worst case scenario is they will simply withdraw their offer of a job and will reconvene the panel with a view to appointing somebody different. You must, therefore, proceed with any negotiation with quiet diplomacy and tact, but at the same time, be confident about what you want to achieve.

Salary

The most frequent source of negotiation is salary. In general terms, individuals moving up the junior hospital doctor ladder should not take a drop in salary. Some appointees have successfully argued that their new salary should be greater not just than their previous basic salary but greater than previous basic *plus* payments for additional duty hours or 'banding' supplement. Some hospitals are more easily won over on this point than others, but whatever the view of a given hospital, you should aim not to accept a drop in your basic annual salary.

The one important exception to this principle is when you move from the end of the specialty training ladder to consultant grade. At this point in the career ladder, there is no formal agreement to protect an individual doctor's salary and it is theoretically possible to lose out. For example, an individual on the top point of the specialist registrar scale, who was receiving a generous number of additional duty hour payments or top 'banding' rate, might find that they are appointed to the bottom increment of the consultant salary scale and subsequently find themselves on a lower salary. This should be resisted, and mindful of the unfair nature of such a move, many hospitals in years gone by adopted a strategy along these lines:

Individuals moving from a specialist registrar (or old-fashioned senior registrar) post into a consultant graded post used to receive one incremental salary point up to a maximum of two increments on the consultant salary scale for demonstrating that they had one or more of the following attributes:

1 They were over the age of 35 years at time of appointment.

2 They held a higher degree, i.e. MD or PhD.
3 They had been in a senior registrar appointment for more than 2 years before promotion to a consultant post.
4 They had previously worked as a locum consultant in their chosen specialty.

These four points were known as the 'unwritten rules' since they did not exist in any generally agreed form nor in any official document. They used to be applied by a large number of hospitals but *not by all*, and nowadays there is very little you can do to demand the application of these old unwritten rules, except negotiation and attempts at gentle persuasion of your future managers. Bear in mind that this issue is now much less relevant following the demise of the senior registrar grade, since trainees tend to be a lot younger than they used to be when they are appointed to their consultant post. All the same, it might be worth senior specialty trainees who have been in post for several years trying to draw attention to the principles behind these rules.

The 'new consultant contract'

In 2004, consultants throughout the United Kingdom moved to a new system of contracts. Instead of a basic working week for consultants being made up of a number of periods of work called 'notional half days', contracts were established based on an agreed job plan, the job plan comprising a number of 'programmed activities' (PAs) some of which are in 'direct clinical care', i.e. clinics, operating theatre sessions, ward rounds and so on, and some of which are considered to be 'supporting professional activity', i.e. time for personal study, audit, research and teaching, etc. The precise terms and conditions of these new contracts varied slightly between appointments to consultant posts in England, Scotland, Wales and Northern Ireland.

There remains a general assumption that the working week for most consultants is based on ten programmed activities, and most hospitals adhere to the original plan that 7.5 'direct clinical care' programmed activities are balanced with 2.5 'supporting' professional activities. But not all hospitals do this, with some trying to impose less favourable terms, for example imposing a ratio of 8 clinical PAs to 2 supporting PAs, or worse still, a ratio of just 9 to 1. This should be resisted by firm negotiation *before* you take up the post. Of course, some consultants are invited to accept contracts based on 11, 12 or even more 'PAs', and that may well be acceptable, since unlike the previous consultant contract, such additional work receives additional salary. It is therefore vital that if you are being appointed to your first consultant post, you make absolutely certain you know and agree the content of your proposed job plan and exactly what remuneration it will attract. Organisations such as the British Medical Association can be extremely helpful in scrutinising a proposed offer of a contract and successful candidates should not hesitate to seek their professional advice before signing anything.

With whom to negotiate?

Negotiation after the interview, and before taking up the offered post, is unlikely to be relevant to most junior doctors. It is, however, often important for new consultants. Discussion of salary should ideally take place with the chief executive of the hospital in which you will be working. There are very few other individuals, with the possible exception of the director of personnel, who have enough power to select the incremental start point of your new salary. You can seek the support of your new colleagues, but it is the managers who will ultimately decide. Remember that most hospital chief executives will be very willing to meet newly appointed consultants, especially so if they were not involved with the appointment process. It is entirely reasonable to request a meeting with this person very shortly after a successful interview. Issues such as salary and removal expenses may be raised at this meeting.

Negotiation about other aspects of your job can often better be done with the clinical director of your new unit or the medical director of the hospital in which you will be working. It is up to these individuals to ensure that you have a balanced, manageable job plan, an adequate office with a reasonable amount of space, a computer and also proper secretarial support. The level of secretarial support will vary from one job to the next but if you are primarily based in a single hospital, perhaps spending no more than a half or 1 day out per week, you should expect to have the services of a full-time secretary. Many hospital managers now view this as an unreasonable luxury but nevertheless it is what you should aim for.

New consultants may feel that there are other aspects of the post which they want to negotiate. For example, if you feel that the job description is totally unreasonable in its demands and expectations, then the time between the offer of the job and your formal acceptance is one possible time to negotiate. Bear in mind, however, that sometimes it is easier and less inflammatory to actually change your pattern of work once you have been performing according to the original job description for a period of several months. Excessively pushy negotiation and obstruction prior to accepting the job offer may simply mean that your future colleagues turn against you and decide to offer the job to someone else.

WHAT IF YOU WEREN'T SUCCESSFUL?

In the opinion of the authors, there is no such thing as 'interview practice', at least not in front of a genuine panel. In previous sections of this book, we have urged that you obtain practice in a mock interview situation with friends and colleagues. The real interview is inevitably a stressful occasion which requires a lot of investment of time and emotion if you are to be successful. Nevertheless, at times in your career you may fail to get the job that you want, and this can be extremely distressing as well as giving rise to a loss of self-confidence. Try to make the best of a bad job and use the experience of an unsuccessful interview as a sort of tool to help you be more successful next time.

Why not write to the panel members and ask them for some feedback? Most members of an interview panel are very happy indeed to speak in general terms about reasons why you were not selected for a job. Remember, however, that the deliberations of an interview panel are totally confidential, so they will not be able to discuss specific issues relating to exactly what was said behind closed doors. All the same, most members of a panel welcome a quiet approach some days after the interview to ask perhaps: 'Were there any questions which I handled particularly badly?' or 'Was there anything on my CV which the panel felt made me unsuitable or inadequately qualified for the job?'

If you know members of the panel particularly well it is also useful to tactfully enquire whether 'they would advise you to continue using the same referees'. It is surprising how often, once prompted with a question such as this, a member of the interview panel will make a gentle suggestion that you, 'consider changing referee number two'. Act immediately if given important information such as this, since it generally suggests that whoever was the second referee has written something seriously damaging to your prospects.

Do not immediately assume that failure in an interview is a 'black mark' on your record, neither should it be considered any form of failure. Often interview panels anguish at great length, deliberating between two and sometimes three names, all of whom they would very much like to appoint to their job and feel rather regretfully that there is only one job to offer. Sometimes, one member of the panel is despatched from the interview room after the result has been announced in order to offer comfort to the unsuccessful candidates. Try not to feel particularly aggrieved if at this stage you are told it was 'within a millimetre' or 'If only we had two jobs you would have got the second one'. It is very easy to retort that 'a miss is as good as a mile', but instead you should bite your lip, keep your immediate thoughts to yourself, and you should try to be encouraged by these warm comments.

CONCLUSION

chapter 18

This book contains a lot of information that we believe will be useful for final-year medical students, junior doctors and also relatively senior doctors who are applying for the next post in their career progression. Bear in mind that it represents one style of dealing with a job application and the process of being interviewed. The style that we have described may not suit everybody, and if you feel that it would not suit you then do not use it. Do not try to pretend that you are someone other than yourself in the interview and do not try to answer questions in a way that seems somehow unnatural to you just because you think you are giving 'the right answers'.

Remember the important key messages stressed elsewhere in this text:

1 Make absolutely sure that you spot the advert in the first place.
2 Find out as much as you can about the interview panel before the interview.

Getting that Medical Job: Secrets for Success, 3rd edition. © Colin J. Mumford and Suvankar Pal. Published 2011 by Blackwell Publishing Ltd.

3 Do not find yourself sitting in an interview for a job that you are not absolutely certain that you want.

4 Throughout the interview remember to try and give an impression of 'cool professionalism with enthusiasm'.

5 Aim to show the interview panel not just that you are 'right for the job' but also that the job is right for you *at this stage in your career*.

If you are unsuccessful do not assume that there is no hope for you and that you are an abject failure. You may have been ranked a close second behind a future Nobel prize winner.

Good luck! There is always an unpredictable side to medical interviews and a degree of luck as well as a great deal of skill is needed. The authors of this book cannot, of course, accept any responsibility whatsoever if things do not work out. Equally, do not blame the authors if you find yourself being unexpectedly successful in obtaining jobs that you had not really intended to get!

INDEX

Getting that Medical Job: Secrets for Success, 3rd edition. © Colin J. Mumford and Suvankar Pal. Published 2011 by Blackwell Publishing Ltd.